Please return/renew this item by the last date shown. Books may also be renewed by phone or internet.

🖥 www3.rbwm.gov.uk/libraries

☎ 01628 796969 (library hours)

☎ 0303 123 0035 (24 hours)

www.rbwm.gov.uk

Royal Borough
of Windsor &
Maidenhead

THE COMPASSION PROJECT

THE COMPASSION PROJECT

A Case for Hope & Humankindness
from the Town that Beat Loneliness

Dr Julian Abel & Lindsay Clarke

aster

An Hachette UK Company
www.hachette.co.uk

First published in Great Britain in 2020 by Aster,
an imprint of Octopus Publishing Group Ltd, Carmelite House,
50 Victoria Embankment, London EC4Y 0DZ
www.octopusbooks.co.uk
www.octopusbooksusa.com

Distributed in the US by Hachette Book Group,
1290 Avenue of the Americas, 4th and 5th Floors, New York, NY 10104

Distributed in Canada by Canadian Manda Group,
664 Annette St, Toronto, Ontario, Canada M6S 2C8

ISBN 978-1-78325-336-4

A CIP catalogue record for this book is available from the British Library.

Printed and bound in the UK.

10 8 6 4 2 1 3 5 7 9

To Carolyn, Bewick, Cerise and Jude

And in memory of Ruth Boswell and Phoebe Clare Clarke

'Compassion is the basis of morality'
Arthur Schopenhauer

'No act of kindness, however small, is ever wasted'
Aesop

'Empathy is the engine that powers all the best in us'
Meryl Streep

'The obvious is often overlooked'
Anon.

CONTENTS

Preface   ix

Introduction   xi

PART ONE

THE WARMTH OF THE HEART:
A Story of Compassion and Community

  1. An Encounter in the Hospital   2

  2. Points of Light   8

  3. A Malnourishment of Compassion   26

  4. The Remedy, or Why Compassion Matters   40

  5. Compassion in Action   54

PART TWO

HARNESSING THE POWER OF COMPASSION

  6. Compassion and the Individual   88

  7. Weaving Compassionate Networks   106

  8. Compassion in General Practice   133

  9. The Wider Reach of Compassionate Action   161

 10. The Politics of Compassion   192

In Conclusion   205

A Manifesto for Compassionate Communities   209

The Compassionate City Charter   215

Acknowledgements   219

Index   221

PREFACE

J ust a few hours before these words were written, thousands of people across the UK opened their doors and windows on empty streets to applaud the dedicated doctors, nurses, carers and auxiliary staff of the healthcare service who are working at the risk of their own health to save lives and protect us all from the alarmingly rapid spread of the Covid-19 virus. Together they are a living manifestation of the active power of compassion, both in individuals and in the community, which is the presiding theme of this book.

The book's main text was written months before the word 'coronavirus' or the term 'social distancing' entered common usage. The grim reality behind those words has now utterly disrupted the customary patterns of our daily life, while causing widespread suffering, grief, anxiety and distress across the world. By revealing the inadequacy of present systems, the pandemic has drawn urgent attention to the need for radical change in the ways we structure and maintain our provision of healthcare and social welfare. To consider what form such change might take is the practical aim and concern of this book, and the gravity of the current crisis strengthens the authors' conviction of its immediate relevance.

The virus has called into question many of the assumptions on which our way of life has been precariously based – not least our sense of invincibility before the natural world. Everyone is susceptible to infection, and survival is guaranteed to no one. The longer-term psychological consequences of such insecurity are unpredictable and will become a matter of serious concern. Yet the virus has also made vividly clear how closely we are connected to one another and how deeply dependent on each other we are. In so doing it has brought forth a remarkable demonstration of the huge resources of humankindness and compassion on which we can call in the hour of need.

By insisting that, in matters that closely affect all our lives, every hour can be an hour of need, this book seeks to make a practical case for hope based on that innate human capacity for compassion as a secure foundational value for a better, more sustainable way of life.

April 2020

INTRODUCTION

**We are probably never more human than when we are
moved by the distress of others.**

S omething new, effective and urgently needed is happening
in the practice of medicine and healthcare. Significant
changes are being brought about not by some recently
discovered wonder-drug but by the practical application of one of
humanity's most valuable assets: the power of compassion.

During a time when social illnesses have become epidemic,
when issues of loneliness have become an urgent murmur at the
failing heart of our communities and the National Health Service
has been under unprecedented pressure, a small town in Somerset
has chosen a different path. With two uncompromising women at
the helm, Dr Helen Kingston and Jenny Hartnoll, along with over
1,000 community connectors, three talking cafés, a Men's Shed and
a Women's Shed, a choir, dozens of peer-support groups and the
28,000 people who live there, Frome's Medical Practice has adopted
an approach to healthcare that has had some rather remarkable
results and brought this small town to the attention of international
news broadcasters, policy makers, strategists and advisors.

In place of the assumption that a pharmaceutical approach
to medicine principally based on combating disease is the route

to health and happiness, the Frome Medical Practice insists that good relationships are the true source of well-being. Not only has it brought the heart back into the community, but it has devised a model that has significantly lowered emergency admissions to hospital. Compassion, it seems, might really be the best medicine after all.

Frome isn't special. It could be any town; it could be your town. And yet the people who live there have a story to tell about the simple, ground-shaking power of compassion that each of us possesses as an innate capacity. If it came in tablet form, it would be hailed as a wonder of modern medicine. By contrast, it's entirely free but offers heartening evidence that when human beings choose to make time for each other, the beneficial effects go far beyond the reach of naive optimism.

How that was done in Frome, and how the town's remarkable achievement carries with it vital choices for the ways in which we might live our own lives, both as individuals and within communities, is the story told in *The Compassion Project*.

PART ONE

THE WARMTH OF THE HEART:

A Story of Compassion and Community

CHAPTER 1

AN ENCOUNTER IN
THE HOSPITAL

S ooner or later, however orderly our lives and no matter how much care we take to keep them secure, for most if not all of us some unanticipated event will shake the very core of our being. The ancient Greek philosopher Heraclitus attributed such events to what he called the *keraunos* – the thunderbolt – which, he declared, steers all things. Its effects can be deeply transformative, but its arrival can take many painful forms – a blow to the heart, the onset of an illness, an accident or injury, a grievous loss or defeat, a breakdown, a bereavement, or some violent convulsion in the world around us. At such stressful times we all need help and solace, and for that we must look to the quality that most defines our humankindness – the power of compassion.

We begin this tale of compassion with the story of two men, good friends, who found themselves separately caught up in and eventually brought together by the challenging ordeals and transformative opportunities that sudden crisis can bring.

One of the men had been living with his wife – she a potter, he a writer – for almost 40 years when, in 2011, she was diagnosed with the onset of dementia. In retrospect, that moment could be perceived as the culmination of a number of incidents – a prolonged series of debilitating migraines, a faint in her pottery studio which caused a severe blow to her head and the subsequent insertion of a pacemaker to control the flow of blood to her brain – but the diagnosis still struck both of them with the shock of the *keraunos*.

Both husband and wife were in their seventies and were now confronted by an irreversible reality which they must face together. So, with the occasional assistance of family and good friends, he became her full-time carer watching over her needs as best he could while medication delayed, but could not prevent, the progress of the disease.

They tried to remain cheerful and philosophical, but two people for whom the power of words had always been important now found it distressingly difficult to sustain a coherent conversation about what was happening to them. And while communication between them stuttered, the world seemed to be closing in around them.

One evening, five years after the original diagnosis, the man found his wife staring into space where she sat, unable to answer when he spoke to her. In the few minutes they had been apart she had suffered a stroke which both impeded her movement and deprived her of the power of speech. Urgently summoned paramedics delivered her to the stroke unit in Bath's Royal United Hospital where, despite the expert tender care she was given, it soon became clear that little could be done to improve her condition – a condition with which, he now feared, he would be unable to cope at home alone.

At that desperate point, he was invited to discuss his anxieties with a kindly discharge nurse. He felt greatly relieved when the nurse offered to arrange for his wife to be transferred to the community hospital in their hometown, Frome. Some of the stress in the situation was eased when she was placed in a private room there, though he remained anxious that this could only be a temporary respite before an eventual move into a nursing home. Then one day he looked up across the room from her bed and, in what felt like a further merciful turn of circumstance, was surprised to see an old friend coming to greet him.

That friend was a doctor who, since his boyhood days, had felt a strong desire to contribute something meaningful to the world. His growing understanding of compassion as a source of greater good had eventually led him to medical school, but while training as a junior doctor in a hospital he had become aware of the dissonance between his own motivating values and much of the practice he observed around him.

Increasingly he found the pressurized culture of hospital life ill-designed to meet the deeper needs of both patients and staff. In 1993, with compassion central to his motivation, he decided to become a specialist in the palliative care of those suffering from terminal illness. Years of working in that field convinced him that one of the most important things he could do to help people approaching the end of their life was to promote, enhance and nourish the capacity for love, laughter and care in the people surrounding the dying patient. After all, he insisted, the principal sources of meaning in our lives are the people we know and love in the places we know and love, which is, of course, why those suffering from terminal illness prefer to be at home with their family as much as possible.

But families cannot cope with everything alone, he realized, and the strain of looking after people as they approach the end of their lives can be severe when only those closest to the person with the illness are involved. But death, dying, loss and care-giving is something we will all experience and when others help – whether this be family, friends, neighbours or the kind-hearted people in our communities – the shared experience transforms the care for everyone involved. The doctor became increasingly involved with a fledgling movement called Compassionate Communities, which began in the field of palliative care and had this approach very much at its heart. During the following years he wrote papers on the theme and was successfully leading regional and national initiatives towards its further development when the *keraunos* struck twice in a single day.

Late in 2015 the hospice in which he worked found itself in dire financial circumstances. As is the case with most charitable institutions, the board of trustees overseeing its services was drawn from members of the business world who had little specific knowledge of, or any expertise in, the true nature of the work it performed. Given the urgent need for a change of management, a new interim chief executive was appointed who decided that the most efficient solution to the hospice's financial problems lay in making severe cuts to staff and services.

That triumph of monetary pragmatism over practical compassion ran directly counter to the spirit of a culture which had been patiently cultivated in the hospice over several years. After several bruising months, the doctor felt driven towards handing in his notice as medical director of the hospice while continuing to perform his clinical work as a consultant. Then, while he was taking a week's leave in which he hoped to recuperate from this blow to his hopes, he received a blunt email from the interim chief executive ordering him not to return to his post. An hour later, while contemplating in a state of shock this cursory end to 15 years of careful work, he answered a phone call to learn that his mother was in a London hospital, diagnosed with terminal leukaemia.

Throughout the next month he travelled back and forth across the country to care for his mother, alongside other members of his family. Using both his skill as a physician and his years of experience with the need for a community of care at such a stressful time, he organized a network of family and friends to give comfort and compassionate support to his mother during her last weeks of life. When she died, she was in a more peaceful and composed state of mind than he had ever previously seen her and the moving experience of keeping her company throughout that time proved both confirmatory and transformative in many ways, both for him and for all involved in that local network of care.

By the time the two men met unexpectedly in Frome's Community Hospital on that October day in 2016, the doctor was working with members of the Frome Medical Practice to create a Compassionate Communities programme in the provision of end-of-life care. Now in close alliance with professional colleagues who shared his values, he was well equipped to give an old friend the advice and guidance he sorely needed during the days when his wife was passing quietly away. He asked gently what was most worrying for his friend, he listened and was able to allay his friend's fears that his wife would have to go into a home. A network of friends and family was engaged to help, and for a man who had never been accustomed to asking for help, simple gestures such as coming to the house for a couple of hours so he could have a restorative walk in the fresh air or the offer of a chat over a pint brought merciful relief to an otherwise overwhelming situation. His strength to look after his wife was restored by their kindness.

In later weeks their conversations moved beyond a mutually affirmative sharing of their recent experience to a fuller recognition of the values and social concerns implicit within it. Both men had endured, in different ways, the impact of the *keraunos.* Their lives had been transformed by it and both recognized that the capacity for active compassion, in themselves and in those who had helped them, had been the deep source of energy driving those changes. Meanwhile, related events already happening in the community around them under the enlightened leadership of the town's medical practice had generated further thought.

The growing collaboration between these two friends led to the writing and publication in *Resurgence & Ecologist* magazine of an article entitled 'Compassion Is the Best Medicine'. They reflected there on the wider implications of the important work being done by Dr Helen Kingston, the lead GP in the Compassionate Frome project, and her team to relate urgent issues of personal health and social welfare to an imaginative programme of community development. Because the results of that work have proved as surprising as they are significant, the article attracted attention worldwide. In consequence, as will already be clear, those friends became the authors of this book.

CHAPTER 2

POINTS OF LIGHT

Compassion, *n*,
The feeling or emotion when a person is moved by the suffering or distress of another, and by the desire to relieve it.

Across the country, and across the world, people of good heart and goodwill are quietly working on imaginative projects to improve the quality of their own lives, the lives of those around them and the world in which they live. Many such initiatives happen in relatively obscure places through the actions of ordinary people outside the usual centres of power who are motivated by that active concern for others which is the hallmark of compassion. Beyond the immediate benefits accruing from their work, those small committed groups may, consciously or unconsciously, be preparing the ground for radical change in the way society as a whole conducts its affairs. They are, in a real sense, encouraging us all to be more fully human.

Inspired by recent events in the life of one small English town, this book sets out the case for the effective restoration of the active power of compassion as a widely available, fundamental force for good in all aspects of human life. In the process, we shall draw attention to research which demonstrates that an innate capacity for compassionate behaviour is so closely woven into the fabric of our bodies that it may not just be metaphorical to speak of compassion as the intelligence of the heart.

Above all, this book insists throughout that to act compassionately is a matter of choice for us all, and that we are free to decide whether or not we want to live in a world where compassion is a fundamental value capable of bringing heartfelt change to the communities in which we live.

Most of us may have a sense of what 'compassion' means, yet, perhaps because of the way it relates an inward urgency of feeling to the need for selfless outward reach, its nature remains somewhat mysterious and difficult to define. To call it 'empathy' doesn't get us very far as it merely replaces a noun derived from Latin with one of Greek origin, as does 'sympathy', which feels too weak to comprehend the warmth and strength of compassion. Yet 'love' seems too large a word to describe an authentic flow of feeling which can happen between people who may know nothing about one another. 'Charity', in its contemporary usage, can, like 'pity', carry an air of condescension. Even a sentence defining compassion as 'participation in another's sorrow', can feel like a reduced account of what is a simultaneous response of the imagination to a motion of the heart that ignites an act of the will. More simply, let's just call it the warmth of the heart.

Every day, a stranger will hurry to the aid of someone who collapses in the street; many will not leave a supermarket without anonymously putting something in the foodbank for those in need and every year people spend time and energy, without thought of personal gain, organizing fundraising events for local, national and international charities. This all offers strong evidence that compassion is deeply intrinsic to human nature – though it is not limited to charitable giving and voluntary work.

Every day, poor people across the world welcome strangers into their homes and offer to share with them what little they have. In contemporary urban life, people often act compassionately in ways so commonly habituated that we don't think of it as compassion. Simply asking about another's health and welfare, the offer of a seat for an older person on a crowded train, helpful guidance to someone who has lost their way, a mother comforting a child not necessarily her own – such mundane examples indicate the degree to which our concern for others and our own dependence on their concern for us are closely woven into the very fabric of our lives.

In *Middlemarch,* George Eliot's great novel of morality and complex human relationships, we are reminded that the Victorians used the word 'compassionate' not only as an adjective to describe a particular quality of feeling, but also as a verb – that is, as the energetic expression of an action. The implication of such usage is that one does not merely *feel* compassion for another person or persons, as one might, for example, while watching a charity appeal on television; rather one is *moved to act* on that feeling, to *compassionate with* the other, to play an active part in addressing their distress. Significantly, that active form of the word has long since dropped out of use and will not be found in the Concise Oxford Dictionary.

An older contemporary of George Eliot, the German philosopher Arthur Schopenhauer, gave much thought to the mysterious nature of compassion. By all accounts he was a cantankerous, self-absorbed man with a pessimistic cast of mind who found it hard to sustain close human relationships. Perhaps for that reason, in his important essay 'The Foundations of Morality', he found it necessary to question why some human beings are prepared to put their own lives at risk in order to save others who are in immediate peril. He asked:

How can it be that the weal and woe of another should directly move my will: that is to say, become my motivation, as though the end served were my own; and even occasionally to such a degree that my own well-being and suffering – which are normally my only two springs of conduct – should remain more or less ignored?

In looking for an answer, he turned to his studies of Eastern traditions of Vedanta and Buddhist philosophy, along with related strains of thought he found in ancient Western philosophy and elsewhere. Together these patterns of thought led him to the metaphysical insight that the plurality of human life is merely illusory 'and that in all individuals of this world – no matter how great their number – there is made manifest only one, single, truly existent Being, present and ever the same in all.' On the basis of this principle he declared that an act of compassionate self-sacrifice occurs 'only because *another* can actually become the final concern of *my* willing', and that 'I can become to such a degree identified with him as to act in a way that annuls the difference between us.'

Of course, no such philosophical speculations are likely to pass through the mind of someone urgently attempting to save another's life, but Schopenhauer offers us an important insight when he thus defines compassion as an act of *imagination* and an effort of the *will* arising from the deep, even unconscious awareness that 'we are all one and the same single Being.' Questions of morality soon merge into issues of metaphysics, and thence into religion, and at the heart of truly religious practice, whatever the faith or denomination, lies the Golden Rule – that one should treat one's neighbour as one would wish to be treated oneself.

But whether we are religious or not, we don't have to engage in metaphysical speculation to see compassion as a quickening motion of the heart that is alive and active in our closest relationships. It's plain enough in a mother's self-denying care for her child, in a son's concern for an elderly parent, or a neighbour's willingness freely to give aid and assistance to someone ill or in distress. On a more far-reaching scale, large secular charities mount major campaigns of relief for famine, earthquakes and other urgent needs every year, and people quickly respond in their millions.

Compassion may begin as a willingness to acknowledge the pain and suffering of others through an act of imaginative identification with that person. This opens the heart into deeper understanding and then prompts the mind to seek ways – however distressing or uncomfortable, and perhaps even dangerous – through which that suffering might be alleviated. When, in our personal and professional lives, the imagination and the will come together in that manner, not only do we cause less harm in the world than might otherwise be the case, we can also have a positive, even transforming impact on those around us and on the wider environment in which we live.

On 25 May 2018, Dr Helen Kingston, a leading GP at Frome Medical Practice, was invited to 10 Downing Street to receive an award for the extraordinary work she and her team had achieved as a result of just such an act of the imagination. Just five years previously, together with her colleague, community development worker Jenny Hartnoll, Helen had created Health Connections Mendip, which became known as the Compassionate Frome project. Its demonstrable success had attracted the attention of her government.

This programme was conceived from the first as an effort to integrate primary healthcare with the creative resources of an activated compassionate community. This was Dr Helen Kingston's vision:

We wanted to create a community where people are supported to be creative, active and resourceful in response to their own and each other's unique and shared needs, with easily accessible integrated care and support available to all.

In so doing, the Compassionate Frome project not only revitalized the life of the town but came up with a practical answer to the notoriously intractable problem of the increasing rate of hospital admissions across the country.

As can be seen, between 2013 and 2017, when the Compassionate Frome project was underway, emergency admissions to hospital in Frome, a town with a population of 28,000 people, were reduced by 14 per cent, while over the same period emergency admissions in Somerset as a whole, which has a population of approximately 500,000 people, went up by 29 per cent.[1]

However, the figures relating to the drop in hospital admissions tend to focus attention on what was, in fact, an unexpected if highly desirable consequence – a happy bonus – of the project's original motivation. Never just about saving money, what the project has shown is that better healthcare and well-being within a community is not about more or better medicine and requires neither disruptive innovations imposed by management nor huge capital investment in staff or technology. It is about taking resources already available in the community – both physical and forces like compassion and goodwill – and connecting them to the people who need them. For the first time, it seems that there is proof that active compassion is unquestionably good not just for people's morale but also for their health and well-being.

---

1 Full details of the published paper can be found in the *British Journal of General Practice*, bjgp.org/content/68/676/e803/tab-article-info

QUARTERLY EMERGENCY ADMISSIONS
FROME AND SOMERSET 2013–2017

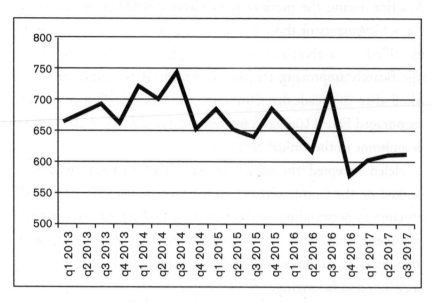

Frome emergency admissions

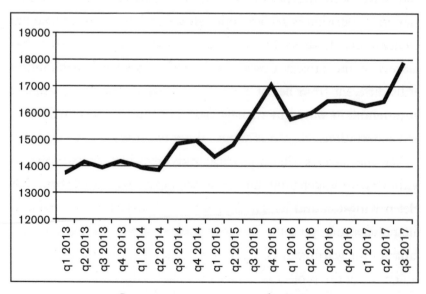

Somerset emergency admissions

The award Helen accepted on behalf of her colleagues was a Points of Light award. This scheme was first introduced in America during the presidency of George W. Bush to recognize the achievements of those many American volunteers – famously identified as 'a thousand points of light' – whose efforts were significantly improving the quality of life in their communities. More than a decade later, in 2014, the success of that scheme encouraged David Cameron's government to develop a partnership programme in the United Kingdom.

Helen accepted the award on behalf of everyone who had worked on the Compassionate Frome project. She said: 'Through a shared understanding of the importance of strong relationships and communities, we have found a way to systematically help individuals to reconnect to their community and establish a sense of agency and belonging.'

A key word in that statement is the plural pronoun 'we'. Helen may have been the person invited to Downing Street, but her modest disposition is accompanied by a quietly firm insistence on accuracy and fairness. She is always quick to point out that the success of the project required the efforts of many people with skills different from her own, and that those people have realized its potential in ways that have far exceeded her own original ideas and expectations.

Yet the success that the project has enjoyed didn't happen without wise leadership, and the leadership given to their team by Helen Kingston and Jenny Hartnoll is an authentic expression of their own strong yet self-effacing characters. They have a particular capacity for warm and caring human relationships of the kind on which the entire project is founded.

A SIMPLE DESIRE BORN OF COMPASSION

At first meeting, Helen Kingston strikes you as the kind of doctor whose calm, good-humoured, quietly sympathetic manner immediately inspires confidence. Her qualities as an alert and sensitive listener, one who knows how to ask the right questions at the right moment, reveal a genuine interest in people as individuals. At the same time, she commands a strongly pragmatic approach to problem-solving based in careful appraisal of the matter in hand. That includes a non-judgmental understanding that a certain comprehensible 'logic' may lie behind the bad choices that people can make in the confusing circumstances of their lives, even though the consequences of those decisions prove harmful to their health and morale. She maintains the firm conviction that when people in such straits are encouraged to work out a different way of relating to their difficulties, they thereby begin to make better decisions and then remarkable transformations can happen.

For Helen, the Compassionate Frome project began simply as a desire to *offer the people she served the best form of health treatment possible.* She had completed her training as a GP with Frome's large medical practice and became a partner there on a job share basis while also working part-time as a clinical assistant in cardiology at the Royal United Hospital in Bath. After becoming a full partner, she joined a smaller team working at Smallbrook Surgery in nearby Warminster where a practice responsible for 4,000 patients was run on a more traditionally modest scale. The patients were known as individuals to a doctor who was reassuringly acquainted with their character and case history, and the receptionist, who had been in place at the surgery for many years, proved to be an invaluable source of information about circumstances that might have a bearing on a patient's individual needs.

The environment of Smallbrook Surgery was congenial, but its medical professionals were still familiar with the experience of witnessing patients suffering from conditions for which the usual protocols of treatment are no true answer, and yet other, more comprehensive means of help are not readily available. These words taken from a piece by Dr Ann Robinson published by the *Guardian* on 14 November 2018 describe that stressful situation well:

> *In my GP surgery this morning, I had nothing to offer a significant proportion of the people I saw. People with lifelong depression, low self-esteem, agoraphobia and anxiety who have become socially isolated. An elderly man and a young mother, both feeling the effects of loneliness and lack of social support. A man in his 60s who has recovered from a heart attack but is finding it hard to motivate himself to overhaul his lifestyle by stopping smoking and starting to exercise and eat healthily. A young man who has back pain for which no specific diagnosis or treatment can be found despite extensive investigations. An elderly, frail lady who is so scared of falling that she's become a prisoner in her own home.*

Such distressing encounters are regrettably common in the surgeries of GPs, as they are often consulted by people dragged deep into the throes of anxiety, depression and thoughts of suicide by unassuageable pangs of loneliness or some other intransigent circumstance of their lives. Doctors are well aware that the care offered by the medical practice may be the only source of close human contact for patients who come to the surgery in this desolate condition. Yet they may have little more than their own stretched resources of sympathy to offer the patient in response, and such knowledge can leave a good doctor uneasy as well as exhausted at the end of the working day.

Faced with the formidable challenges of a GP's life, Helen did what she could for patients suffering from anxiety, depression and other behavioural problems by using savings made from the prescriptions budget to refer them to the local health trainer employed at Smallbrook Surgery – someone who works individually with people to help them develop healthier lifestyles – and other related public health services. But she was increasingly aware that the procedures of a typical surgery-based consultation are not by themselves effective in bringing about truly life-enhancing changes. So what might be a viable alternative?

Let us return to Helen's vision. She had in mind a view of 'a community where people are supported to be creative, active and resourceful in response to their own and each other's unique and shared needs, and there is easily accessible and integrated care and support available to all.' Such an approach would be less specifically targeted than the limited number of supervised sessions her team could offer. Much stronger therapeutic benefits would be achieved by engaging patients in lively relationships with other people through activities, which would strengthen their personal and social confidence and thus help them to find their own solutions to the problems that troubled them.

It was evident, however, that such a programme would require the building of an interactive network of compassionate community resources, made up of both individuals and groups, who could support the transformation of individual patient's lives. For that, additional staff with the right skills of social organization would be needed and there was no scope in the Smallbrook practice's limited budget to risk the cost of recruiting them.

The disparity between Helen's imaginative vision of what ought to be possible and the constraints limiting her scope for action became increasingly frustrating. But when confronted with an un-met need,

Dr Helen Kingston feels compelled to meet it and she remained unfazed by apparently intractable problems. Then, in 2013, an opportunity to act in the way she had in mind presented itself nearby in Frome, where innovative developments were already happening.

In a process that was to become known as 'flatpack democracy', a coalition known as Independents for Frome had begun to wrest control of the town council from the traditional political parties. Their focus was firmly fixed on effective action in response to local needs and on the revitalization of the town's community life. Here, in a place Helen already knew well, her vision might be realized.

Set around a bend of the river for which it was named and surrounded by slopes of lush pasture where sheep might safely graze, Frome in Somerset was once a thriving centre of the woollen industry and more important in its day than Manchester. The fine Grade II listed houses built by the weaving masters of the town are evidence of the wealth they enjoyed, while ranks of attractive stone cottages in the narrow streets once housed the forebears of Frome's still largely working-class population. The iron ore found and worked in the surrounding combes contributed to local prosperity by providing raw material for a metal-casting business that survived well into the twentieth century and produced some of London's prominent statuary, including *Boadicea and Her Daughters* on the Thames' Victoria Embankment and *Lady Justice* on top of the Old Bailey law courts. There was once a silk mill here and a large print works.

Some of the buildings that recall the town's busy industrial past have been repurposed, sometimes converted into gallery space or craft workshops, while others are brownfield sites awaiting development. The town's impressive number of ancient inns and non-conformist chapels also bears witness to what had been a lively community. But like many other small market towns across England,

Frome was left high and dry by the northward shift of energy that came with the Industrial Revolution. Through various economic recessions and recoveries the town has been reinventing itself ever since, and recent years have seen a considerable improvement in its fortunes. Walk down the high street today and you will encounter many independent shops and bustling cafés, and from March to December, on the first Sunday of every month, there is the Frome Independent Market, devoted to local traders, craft makers and artists. It's like any other town, but it has found its spirit once again.

A major new development came in 2013 when Frome's large medical practice was moved out of a 1960s dilapidated single-storey building, next to a Victorian hospital building, into a spaciously designed health centre. The appearance of this impressive complex within easy reach of the town centre immediately aroused expectations of a commensurate improvement in the services on offer – more doctors and nurses to staff the fine buildings, and shorter waits than had long been the case for appointments and treatment. However, in a time of prolonged economic austerity and tight budgets, it was not going to be easy to meet such reasonable expectations. Nevertheless, Helen Kingston made the move from her congenial but circumstantially limited work at Smallbrook Surgery to re-join the much larger group practice in Frome. What she had in mind for the town would bring about changes of a different, more wide-ranging and radical order.

Around that time, plans were afoot to replace the funding of single medical practices across Somerset by a Clinical Commissioning Group (CCG). These opportunities blossomed because of a strong financial position of the CCG under the leadership of David Slack. This enabled a culture of devolved leadership and innovation. Trust was given and resources enabled to develop without micromanagement. Frome Medical Practice was also gifted a federation manager, Michael Bainbridge, with a background in social care who shared Helen's ethos and gave the support and crucially also the freedom to make this happen.

Alert to the opportunities this might create, Helen applied for the funding to begin developing a model that she believed would change medical practice, and her bid proved successful.

She was now a trusted partner in a large and supportive practice that serviced a population of around 30,000 people and was underpinned by funding strong enough to take the manageable risk of employing the additional staff member – on behalf of all the GP surgeries in the Mendip area of Somerset – who was needed to put her energetic programme of community-based healthcare into action. Meanwhile, another woman with a related vision of her own was already active in and around Frome.

For family reasons, Jenny Hartnoll had recently moved westwards from Harlesden, a district of London once notorious as the gun crime capital of the UK, where she had successfully set up charities, motivated other collaborative groups and organized imaginative events to improve the quality of life in that hard-pressed area. She arrived in Somerset in 2006 hoping to secure a post which would give her scope to continue to do that kind of work.

Unfortunately, no such post was on offer. But she had to make a living, so eventually took a job with the Somerset Partnership's health training service. As a trainer, she would meet eight people a day for six weekly one-to-one sessions in which she worked to help them set achievable targets and reach their own goals of healthy lifestyles. In so doing, the anxieties and depression caused by their various debilitating disorders improved.

Jenny Hartnoll has an optimistic, approachable nature well equipped to encourage the efforts of people in such difficult straits, but her years of work in some of the toughest districts of London had shown her how improved social connections can reach deeply into the needs of depressed and lonely people by reducing their feelings of isolation and helping them gain the confidence to take more positive control of their lives. This was particularly inspired in her work with Open Age, a charity devoted to keeping people fit and active, both physically and mentally, in North Kensington. Surely such initiatives should be possible in Somerset, too?

Jenny observed that Frome differed from the rest of the county in that many of its referrals to the health training programme came not through GPs but from word-of-mouth contact with friends and neighbours. This suggested a lively pattern of goodwill and mutual concern in the way Frome people talked to each other. That convivial spirit was further evidenced by the large number of clubs, societies, creative organizations and charities already active in the town. Here were resources waiting to be tapped, yet when she proposed to use the experience she had gained in London by setting up support groups rather than just working with individuals and by engaging the existing life of the community in her work she was met with little encouragement. Though her sense of frustration increased, Jenny drew upon her innate belief in doing something about the problems she encountered rather than merely complaining about them.

To her experienced eye, what was missing in the community life of Frome was a centralized place where information about its various activities could be collated in a publicly available directory. This would alert people to the existence of the range of available resources, relate them to one another and sharpen the town's awareness of its own vitality. Like Helen Kingston, Jenny regards a deficiency less as a matter of regret than as an incentive to act, and here was work that could be done.

On her own initiative, in her own time and in her own kitchen, she began to research and collect all the information she could find about what was happening in and around Frome. Then, in 2011, she proceeded to organize events under the title GO FROME and develop a web directory. The primary aim of the project was simply to advertise as widely as possible the many uplifting experiences freely available around the town.

In a sense, what Jenny had pointed out was obvious, yet no one in the town had thought to act in quite this way before, and her efforts to alert the community of Frome to the extensive range of its own resources met with enthusiastic response. In particular, the wider implications of her work were well understood by the partners at the health centre, who asked to meet her.

On the night before the meeting, heavy snow fell on the town, which meant Jenny had to walk to get to the health centre. Flustered and dishevelled, she turned up late for the appointment, thinking she must cut an unimpressive figure in her snow-covered coat under what she worried was the impatient gaze of a team of busy doctors. During the conversation, she caught the eye of a woman sitting across from her and felt a strong sense of connection.

Sometime later, she was back working full-time as a health trainer when her eye was caught by a job advertisement in the local press. Placed by the medical practice, it sought applicants for a post combining the skills and experience of a community development worker with those of a website designer. Dismayed that her limited IT skills left her disqualified for a job that would otherwise have suited her perfectly, she put it aside. But the more she thought about it, the more strongly she felt that the practice would be very lucky to find anybody with that unlikely combination of skills.

By the time she decided to go for the job the date for applications had expired, but she called to ask if a late response might be acceptable. The answer came that it was. An interview was arranged at which she turned up well prepared to describe her ideas for a scheme which would help patients dealing with long-term conditions to live more independent and empowered lives. The scheme would set up scores of mutual support groups to bring together people who were recovering from the same condition – for example, strokes, chronic lung disease, macular degeneration along with other debilitating illnesses. Once fully developed, this would become a network of advice and support for patients, carers and the wider community, which would improve the general well-being of patients as well as overcoming the social isolation that tended to afflict both them and the people whose lives were restricted by the need to care for them.

What Jenny had presented was effectively a three-year plan of things that could and should be done as part of the town's medical service, but the position had been advertised as only a single-year appointment. She was well aware of this as she walked away from the interview and wondered whether her proposals were just too ambitious. Then her phone rang and she was astonished to be told that the job was hers.

Much later she was told that the interview had been a virtual formality. Dr Helen Kingston, the person with whom Jenny felt she had made contact at the first meeting, and who was the prime mover behind the medical practice's approach, had been deeply disappointed when Jenny failed to respond to the advertisement – it had in fact been placed specifically to attract her. She had therefore been hugely relieved when her late application arrived.

SEEDS OF COMPASSION

Jenny Hartnoll, who has an unshakeable trust in synchronicity as a creative force, must have been convinced that she and Dr Kingston were destined for each other. Both women are resolute, pragmatic and unassuming. They are both deeply serious in their dedication to strong humanitarian values, while sharing a lively sense of humour. They may have come from different professional backgrounds – Helen's in medicine, Jenny's in community development – but just as they have come together in friendship, so their fruitful partnership over succeeding years has created a vital bond between primary care and the welfare of communities. Jenny says, 'What I was doing already was in line with what Helen had in mind. I somehow knew I was going to work in Frome Medical Practice. When I met Helen, we knew we were on the same pathway.'

Neither Helen nor Jenny would claim to be anything out of the ordinary, but each speaks of the other as someone rather special. They have a mutually supportive relationship that brings out the strengths in each of them. However, both are quick to stress that many people – all of them points of light – have played a vital role in the project's success, often in coincidentally inventive ways that neither of them could have anticipated.

The results of this inspirational work would eventually bring to this small Somerset town a bevy of prime ministerial advisors, strategists from the NHS, journalists from the national media and a camera team from Swedish TV, along with researchers from widespread foreign parts and representatives of medical practices across the country and abroad, all of them keen to observe what has been happening in Frome and to learn from it. A flow of inspirational stories arrives constantly from other parts of the United Kingdom, Australia and New Zealand, among others. As Jenny says, 'The neural pathways not just in the community, but across the world, are beginning to light up.'

CHAPTER 3

A MALNOURISHMENT
OF COMPASSION

'As you get older your whole life changes. Your children have grown up and gone, and I can't expect anyone to keep coming here to see me when they've got their own lives to lead. I don't think anyone can explain what the loneliness is like. I was in a terrible state. I knew that if I didn't get somebody to see me that I would die.'

Sue, resident of Frome

Medical practitioners have long been troubled by the debilitating sequence of events that commonly occurs when patients fall sick. The illness causes fatigue. Fatigue affects mobility with an accompanying decline in both the energy and motivation to leave the house. The will to do such domestic tasks as cooking and cleaning weakens. So too the readiness to drive and go about the business of making a living. Such inertia leads to social isolation and, with it, a diminishing sense of self-worth. In such depleted circumstances one's sense of identity begins to blur. Soon one may begin to wonder whether there's any point remaining on this earth.

Loneliness is frequently the cause as well as the effect of such decline. It's what too easily happens when ailing people lack the surrounding presence of a caring network of support and it has become so loud a murmur at the heart of our failing communities that the British government has found it necessary to appoint a minister for loneliness with the specific responsibility for remedying the situation. Whether administrative measures put in place by politicians far removed from the harsh realities of life on the streets are the best way of responding to a social crisis that blights the lives of far too many people is among the questions that this book will raise.

What is certainly the case is that increasing numbers of otherwise healthy people suffer from a disabling sense of loneliness and a consequent loss of self-esteem. It figures among the causes of long waiting lists for appointments with a doctor and too often it creates critical conditions which result in emergency admission to hospital. Meanwhile, research has also shown that chronic loneliness increases the risk of early death by 20 per cent.

The urgent health concerns of the old and sick are not the only symptoms of a failure of compassion at the heart of our communities. In 2019, a poll conducted by YouGov for the Prince's Trust found that 18 per cent of more than 2,000 young people who submitted responses did not agree with the statement that 'Life is really worth living'. That figure doubled the number who had made the same admission ten years earlier. In the same poll, 27 per cent of the responders disagreed with the statement 'I feel my life has a sense of purpose', while nearly 50 per cent admitted to a sense of inadequacy when they compared their lives with others on social media. Such expressions of anxiety and desperation feel consistent with reports of an increase in the number of teenagers taking their own lives and others injured or dying of knife crime.

WHERE DID OUR COMPASSION GO?

For centuries, poets, novelists, artists and philanthropists have been calling our attention to the consequences of a lack of compassion, yet still, in an era where people might be more prosperous and comfortable than in any preceding it, such disturbing statistics confront us with an image of a deeply troubled and disconsolate society. At this moment we are living in a time when far too many young people – those in whom our best hopes for the future should lie – are suffering from solitary pangs of anxiety and defeat, along with far too many old and lonely men and women who find themselves bereft of the enlivening sense of value and meaning which caring relationships bring.

In much the same way that the proliferating need for food banks in one of the world's richest countries bears witness to an inequitably applied regime of economic austerity, those bleak responses to the questions of the YouGov poll are symptomatic of a culture now suffering from a chronic malnourishment of compassion. An examination of how this state of affairs has come about may help us to a better understanding of how an adequate remedy might be found. But it will first require a hard – if highly condensed – look at some of the darker aspects of recent social and economic history in which that sickness thrived.

Whatever the major religions of the world have urged us to do by way of the Golden Rule, long centuries of almost ceaseless fighting for power, land and riches on the one hand and the bitter struggle for survival on the other have rarely found space to include in their headlines the vital importance of compassion. In that respect the current era differs little from others. But what must surely be different is the staggering fact that, of the almost 8 billion people presently living on Earth, the overall beneficiaries of those age-old struggles are the 26 men who now control as much of the world's wealth as do the poorest 50 per cent.[2]

Of course, there has always been inequality and injustice, especially where the distribution of wealth is at stake, but if there has ever been a time when so vast a gap in prosperity has existed between so many and so few, it surely lacked the degree of consciousness of that disparity which is now available to us. We know that it's the case, we know that it need not be the case, and that the dire conditions of poverty in which so many people are forced to live are the direct consequence of our failure to act responsibly on that knowledge. Yet we persist in our all but mesmerized assent to unsustainable patterns of behaviour which, as well as causing needless misery to millions, are also devastating the natural order of the planet on which our lives depend. At the same time, though less visibly, they may be doing comparable damage to our souls. For it seems to be the case that, however desirable the material benefits of luxury, comfort and convenience that have been afforded to many people, the last three centuries, since the onset of the Industrial Revolution, have also had significantly corrosive effects on human sensibilities.

In *The Amber Spyglass*, the third book of *His Dark Materials*, Philip Pullman offers a powerful metaphor for this state of things. He describes there how a scientist who has been transported to another world in another universe makes a device – the amber spyglass of the title – which allows her to see clearly what would otherwise remain invisible. When she looks through it she sees particles of that glowing dust which she understands is the stuff of life – that which gives us the power to love and learn to be compassionate. But in the oppressed world she inhabits, that dust is leaking out of the universe.

2 Information taken from the Oxfam report *An Economy for the 99%* by Deborah Hardoon (Oxfam International, January 2017; DOI: 10.21201/2017.8616).

THE INDUSTRIALIZATION OF HUMANITY

In the rapidly changing world of the early nineteenth century, the Romantic poets – including William Blake, who would become an inspirational figure for Pullman – saw that the newly mechanized mode of industrial life would have harmful effects on the quality of human life and culture. Far from being fanciful inhabitants of some ivory tower, they knew that the mills and factories of northern England were first funded by profits from the Atlantic slave trade – a systematic relegation of large numbers of human beings to the sub-human status of animals and chattels – which required the extinguishing of all sense of compassion. They also foresaw that the movement of workers into cities and towns, away from close contact with the rhythms of the natural world, would inevitably break the bonds of ancient communities and coarsen the minds and hearts of those who were put to the iron service of machines. The new science brought about a sceptical materialism, which reduced the once sacred status of the natural world to an inanimate realm of exploitable matter.

Old superstitions were called into question by these developments but, as A N Whitehead stated almost a century ago, 'The doctrine of minds, as independent substances, leads directly not merely to private worlds of experience, but also to private worlds of morals,' thus freeing rugged individualists to exploit opportunities opened by a limited moral outlook. Consciously or otherwise, these philosophical assumptions were among the power sources of the Industrial Revolution, and if life in the rural world had always been hard for the disenfranchised poor in many ways it became still harsher in the grim environment of the towns and cities.

Some philanthropic industrialists, mostly Quakers, took steps to improve the lot of their workers, and their campaigns against the worst excesses led to limited measures of reform. More radical thinkers such as Marx and Engels (the son of a textile manufacturer) would demand revolutionary change, but deference to established power and enforced acceptance of rigorous social divisions – for which divine authority was claimed – remained the general rule. In such a world, there was little light and clean air for the delicate flower of compassion to prosper.

Meanwhile, the need for the raw materials of industry and the creation of new markets gave further impetus to the expansion of empire. Coal was plentiful at home but minerals, rubber, oil, cotton and other essentials had to be found abroad, mostly in lands inhabited by people who were conveniently regarded as savages (that is, sub-human) and were therefore considered eligible for subjection and, in some cases, extermination. Much of Britain's imperial history is far from glorious in this respect, and the assumption that 'the manifest destiny' of the United States led westwards allowed a nation, which had been founded on slavery, to practise virtual genocide on the indigenous peoples of the continent. Such atrocities lend credence to the assertion that evil will be quick to enter the space left empty by a heart vacant of compassion and the following century would offer further proof.

THE WAR ON COMPASSION

The Great War of 1914–1918 was an industrially armed clash between imperial nations, and that it cost the lives of many thousands of men in callously planned, inconclusive battles is common knowledge. Yet its consequences were such as to make a second world war inevitable – a war which witnessed genocide on an industrial scale and eventually climaxed with the total destruction of large cities by the devastating power of nuclear weaponry. Nor was that the end of an atrociously violent century in which powerful nations later preferred to fight their wars in regions far from their homelands.

Belatedly, we have now come to recognize the traumatizing effects of warfare on the soldiers and civilians directly caught up in its ravages. But there is also a very real sense in which, at more or less deeper levels, none of us escapes unscathed from such widespread recourse to violence. So-called compassion fatigue is one of its more shameful symptoms, for, as Seamus Heaney said in his Nobel Prize acceptance lecture, 'Every day, as we channel-surf over so much live coverage of contemporary savagery,' we are left 'highly informed but nevertheless in danger of growing immune, familiar to the point of over-familiarity with old newsreels of the concentration camp and the gulag.'

The successful prosecution of any war requires a massive effort of shadow-projection – the failure to acknowledge and assimilate the darkness in our own minds and hearts because it is easier to attribute it all to the enemy, to demonize them, to think of them as rats or 'gooks' rather than as human beings who are as vulnerable as ourselves. To do that, one must wilfully withhold all impulses of compassion. Yet that withholding is itself a form of psychological damage. By confining us inside a world where the prevailing story is that of *us* against *them*, it increases suspicion and fear and hardens our hearts in ways that can only leave us feeling less rather than more secure. In such a culture, shows of feeling, especially by men, are often read as signs of weakness. The result is that we become more prone to defend ourselves by a competitive stance against the possible threats we perceive around us; more protective of what we believe to be our own interests and more fearful of the future.

Even as prosperity returned after the Second World War, such sentiments as 'look after number one' and 'I'm all right, Jack' had already entered common parlance. That state of heart and mind is the exact opposite of the sense of human unity which saints and philosophers have claimed to be the ground of our being and our morality, and the cumulative effect of many people behaving that way aggravates the malnourishment of compassion in the world.

COMMERCE OVER COMPASSION

Nor are wars and violence the sole contributors to that condition. In 1928, Edward Bernays, a nephew of Sigmund Freud, published a book titled *Propaganda* that would have a significant impact on general human welfare by its advocacy of the deliberate creation of public demand for the products put on sale by commercial interests. Bernays asserted that:

> *The conscious and intelligent manipulation of the organized habits and opinions of the masses is an important element in democratic society. Those who manipulate this unseen mechanism of society constitute an invisible government which is the true ruling power of our country. We are governed, our minds are moulded, our tastes formed, our ideas suggested, largely by men we have never heard of... A single factory, potentially capable of supplying a whole continent with its particular product, cannot afford to wait until the public asks for its product; it must maintain constant touch, through advertising and propaganda, with the vast public in order to assure itself the continuous demand which alone will make its costly plant profitable...If we understand the mechanism and motives of the group mind, is it not possible to control and regiment the masses*

according to our will without their knowing about it? The recent
practice of propaganda has proved that it is possible.

American politicians eagerly embraced this commercial approach
to meaning and value by exhorting people to go and buy more of
such luxury goods. In 1929 (shortly before the Wall Street crash) a
report issued by a committee set up by President Hoover to assess
recent economic change proclaimed: 'Economically we have a
boundless field before us; there are new wants which will make way
endlessly for newer wants, as fast as they are satisfied.'

This plan to create dissatisfaction and stimulate people's desire
to buy things which they did not actually need was the birth of
the sales and marketing industry. Since then it has become ever
more sophisticated in finding ways to maximize the profits of
international corporations, often without concern for the impact
on the general welfare of people or the environment in which they
live. The crazy scrambles to grab bargains on Black Friday and in
January sales provide graphic images of the way that stimulation
of the need to define our identity by the things we possess has
affected our values and our moral welfare. The same might be said
of the cynical energy put into television advertising by the gambling
industry and the ubiquitous use of sexual imagery to encourage
spending on what are thus made to seem desirable goods.

More visibly, the effects of advertising also reach into our health.
The tobacco industry was a historical marker in the wilful ignoring
of responsibility for the damage it does to countless lives. And too
many companies within the pharmaceutical industry – whose reason
for existence is supposedly to benefit humanity – have falsified
drug trials, destroyed the reputations of academics who oppose
their methods, cleverly advertised their wares and paid individual
health practitioners to prescribe their products while suppressing

information about possible harmful effects. Almost every major pharmaceutical company has received fines of hundreds of millions of dollars for such criminal activity with little significant effect on their willingness to change their ways. Even research – supposedly objective in its analysis of cause and outcome – is sometimes so influenced by this process that, as a matter of routine, peer reviewed scientific journals now ask for statements concerning conflicts of interest created by sources of funding and payment.

The depths to which pharmaceutical companies will stoop can be seen in the roots of the opioid epidemic in the United States. Between 2011 and 2017, cases of synthetic opioid (pharmaceutically manufactured morphine-like substances developed for medical pain relief) overdose rose from one per thousand to nine per thousand. During the same six-year period, drug overdose deaths rose from 20,000 to 50,000. Insys Therapeutics, producers of a synthetic opioid that can be delivered through a nasal spray, were found guilty of bribing doctors to overprescribe the medication that resulted in opioid addiction. This behaviour was unfortunately not limited to Insys Therapeutics alone. Johnson and Johnson were fined $465 million (although the verdict of this case is under appeal) and two other pharmaceutical companies came to agreements with state prosecutors. Two further companies received fines of $270 million and $85 million. A more complete description of the wide variety of techniques and strategies used by pharmaceutical companies can be found in the book *Deadly Medicines and Organized Crime* written by Peter Gotzsche, a highly regarded pharmacologist. Even within the pharmaceutical industry, companies are prepared to behave in a way that results in thousands of deaths.

Meanwhile, close links between large corporations and politicians are carefully cultivated as individuals flow between the two groups. Such partnerships provide political funding and, in return, company advisors are afforded places in key decision-making bodies. This is now a normal process and, by such subtle means of manipulation, profitability is expanded while compassion, which should be a prevailing value at the heart of the health industry, is reduced to mere tokenism.

Nor is it just our bodily health which can suffer from industrialized commercial processes. In his powerful book, *The Master and His Emissary*, Iain McGilchrist shows that the material advantages brought by science and technology come at an unanticipated price. The exponential speed with which their power has advanced in recent decades has created an increasingly worrying imbalance in the way our minds tend to operate. In consequence, we become ever more reliant on the left brain, with its capacity for cold, abstract, analytic thought, at the expense of the right hemisphere of the brain, which provides an essential countervailing source of meaning, context and value – each of which is an element vital to the proper functioning of the compassionate imagination.

DIGITAL REVOLUTION

Digital technology is the direct product of left-brain thought processes and, since the beginning of the century, it has brought about significant changes in both individual behaviour and social relations. Those changes are now so profound that they amount to a critical disjunction between the present and the relatively recent past. The sight of people with one hand to their faces walking the streets urgently talking to someone who isn't there without taking much notice of what is happening around them may be an unremarkable feature of everyday reality for younger members of society, but to an elderly person, such a disregard for the civilities of public behaviour is a social aberration.

Such an everyday example of the way left-brain ingenuity alters human relations may seem to overstate the harmful effects of what can be seen as a desirable means of communication. The prevalence of left-brain thinking results in a corrosion of both moral and aesthetic sensibility with a failure to pay attention to compassion, and the evidence for it can be seen almost everywhere. This results in the loss of a sense of consequences of actions, such as the digitized financial dealings which have had a disastrous economic impact across the globe; in online crime and the corruption of electoral procedures; in unemployment caused by the robotization of workplaces; and perhaps most alarmingly, in the accelerating creation of artificial intelligence. More widely, it now manifests in the personal lives of countless people as a preference for the ever-proliferating seductions of virtual reality over the warm, pheromonic contact of immediate human interaction.

Major changes to the built environment have also had socially harmful consequences. In many urban areas, the streets, where a variety of shops and small businesses used to flourish, while chatter, childcare and incidental crime-watch were the usual order of the day, have now been demolished and replaced by urban motorways and high-rise tower blocks, both of which are inimical to any fluent sense of community life. At the same time, our social world has become increasingly atomized and cut off from the natural environment which it despoils, yet on which its existence depends.

In the workplaces of the land, skills which people may have spent half a lifetime developing are abruptly made redundant and businesses are rendered subject to fiercely competitive market forces over which they have little or no control. Even national governments find themselves relatively impotent since the multinational operation of speculative capitalism now makes, in its own interests, the impersonal decisions which determine the prevailing realities of the global economy.

Meanwhile, when they are not being targeted by a battery of examinations in school, children can quickly become addicted to virtual meetings with friends and strangers on their screens, sometimes suffering bullying. One way or another, both they and their parents or carers are caught up in a struggle to keep pace with changes that have already confined many elderly people to uncomprehending cultural exile. As recent political activity online has shown, it's also a world in which that elusive phenomenon, the truth of things, is up for grabs and largely determined by whichever newspaper, TV channel or social echo chamber you may choose to credit.

AND YET, THERE IS KINDNESS IN THE AIR

Fortunately, this dismal picture is not, of course, the whole story. As was indicated earlier, the capacity for compassion is still to be found to a greater or lesser extent, either positively active or deeply embedded, in all of us, and however bitter the lessons of history may be, we human beings are as much the case for hope as we are the authors of our own despair.

Such projects as that of Frome's successful attempt to build a Compassionate Communities programme strongly argue the case for hope, and there are many of them actively working for change across the country and abroad. Significantly, such projects arise from local grassroots in response to immediately felt need, rather than being imposed from above by some impersonal ideology. And the problems facing the town of Frome are similar in essence to those faced by other villages, towns and cities across the United Kingdom, although these problems may have a different emphasis, intensity and severity than those in Frome.

As we will hear, many heartwarming stories have come out of Frome – acts of simple kindness and compassion from daily existence that are a natural part of community members spending time with each other. The Compassionate Frome project built on this fundamental kindness, spreading it widely across the community. So, what is the Pullmanesque 'dust' that powers them? The next chapter will consider the vital constituents – biological and social, ethical and spiritual – which together might provide a revitalizing remedy for that disabling state of malnutrition which not only afflicts the health and welfare of the lonely and the depressed but also that of the many hard-pressed communities in which they live.

CHAPTER 4

THE REMEDY, OR WHY
COMPASSION MATTERS

Five years ago I had a stroke. After I came out of hospital, I sat and felt sorry for myself for a while. After three or four months my wife had had enough of it and we split up. I felt totally alone. Coming to the shed totally changed my life. I did get to the point of considering whether life was worth it anymore. Then I remembered my grandson and that stopped me from going any further and made me do something about it. The shed was the place where it worked. It's given me back my self-confidence. It has given me a load of new friends and I now get involved in voluntary projects – something I never would have dreamed of before. There are a few people here I can just pick up the phone to and say, 'Are you doing anything?' They say no, just come on round. I haven't had friends like that for a long time.

Steve, interviewed for the Swedish TV programme
Korespondentern as part of a documentary about
the Frome project

The Compassionate Frome project first attracted serious national and international attention because in one vital aspect it was unique: here was the first project to record a measurable reduction in emergency admissions to hospital across a population. Though that wasn't the scheme's only achievement, it was certainly important because it offered a potential answer to the seemingly insoluble problem confronting Western health services.

Over the previous two decades, the UK government had sought to reduce public reliance on the hospitals, which are the most expensive part of the health service, by instituting a policy of 'care in the community'. But year after year this policy failed because it placed an unmanageable degree of stress on local medical practices and thus paradoxically increased the demand for emergency care at the hospitals. In winter months, under an onslaught of emergency arrivals, a national health service which has been hailed internationally as a triumph of civilization teetered towards disaster.

The increase in the number of admissions to hospital was unpredictable from day to day, and wards were routinely opened and closed to cope with fluctuating demand. When a ward is closed, the team working there is disbanded and the staff is laid off. But a renewed rise in demand means that the ward has to be reopened. Staff from other wards have to cover it, which weakens the team on their own ward. It then takes considerable time to create the new team, so in both wards there may be a decline in the quality of care, meaning that patient safety is affected. When an epidemic crisis hits, routine operations have to be postponed to make available the requisite number of beds.

By January 2018, the accumulated stress on hospitals had become so severe that, across England, all routine operations were cancelled. The immediate effect was to lengthen waiting lists, which had the knock-on effect of worsening the condition of the waiting patients, thus complicating their eventual treatment. This cycle of opening and closing wards, which happens in English hospitals year after year, not only puts safety of care at risk, it significantly increases costs.

Such problems are not confined to the English National Health Service, so it's small wonder that, once the results announced by the Frome experiment had been subjected to statistical evaluation, they were warmly welcomed both at home and abroad. Health professionals and politicians were eager to know what apparent magic Frome had worked, and what the vital transformative link between an energetic programme of community development and an improved provision of local healthcare might be. The answer was compassion.

SOCIAL RELATIONSHIPS AND HUMAN HEALTH

We have seen how, in trying to account for self-sacrificial acts of compassion, the philosopher Schopenhauer drew on the insight that each human life exists in a unified sea of consciousness. It feels consistent with that view of things that when a new development surfaces in a particular place, it will soon come to be seen as an early manifestation of a shift in perspective that has also been emerging elsewhere. Not surprisingly, therefore, Dr Helen Kingston, Jenny Hartnoll and their team were not the only people actively exploring the connection between individual health and that of the wider community.

A team at the Brigham Young University in Utah had previously been conducting a programme of research which turned up some very interesting results.

The leader of that programme, Professor Julianne Holt-Lunstad, described her work in these terms:

My program of research examines the influence of both the quantity and the quality of social relationships on long-term health and on risk for mortality, and the biological pathways (e.g., cardiovascular, neuroendocrine, genetic) by which such associations may occur. I also consider the potentially detrimental influence of negativity in close relationships (e.g., ambivalence, marital distress). My studies have examined social relationships at a network level, among married couples, in mother-and-infant relationships, and within friendships. My work is interdisciplinary and takes a multimethod approach including experimental, naturalistic, meta-analytic, and intervention studies.

In 2010, she and her research team published a paper titled 'Loneliness and Social Isolation as Risk Factors for Mortality: A Meta-Analytic Review'. Having examined a wide variety of interventions in order to compare their impact on the risk of dying, the paper confirmed what was already known – that good social relationships are fundamental to human health. More significantly, however, it also concluded that the impact of such a benevolent context is more effective than any other kind of preventative strategy. Remarkably, the accumulated evidence showed that good social relationships have a greater effect on extending length of life than do such measures as giving up smoking or drinking alcohol, maintaining a healthy diet, taking regular exercise, weight loss or the treatment of high blood pressure.

Those findings are as important as they are unexpected because they show that we can actually do more for our health by improving the quality of our relationships with the world around us than by making any other change we know. Yes, we may have to call on other interventions for the treatment of existing conditions, but the most effective *preventative* medicine at our disposal – the remedy which is most likely to increase the number of years we can hope to live – is the creation and preservation of good social relationships. This would become the foundation of Dr Helen Kingston's vision for providing health and social care for the community of Frome. Reinforcement of Holt-Lundsted's encouraging conclusions can be found in Susan Pinker's book *The Village Effect: Why Face-to-Face Contact Matters.* She writes there that, 'Few see looking after others as therapeutic for the person who does the caretaking or consider community involvement as therapeutic as drugs. Yet there is mounting evidence that a rich network of face-to-face relationships creates a biological force field against disease.' Pinker's book examines in detail how social relationships have a direct effect on health by drawing together evidence from a wide variety of sources to demonstrate that face-to-face communication is the key component in improving length of life and general well-being.

THE WARMTH OF YOUR HEART PREVENTS YOUR BODY FROM RUSTING

A clear, and now much-studied, demonstration of this evidence can be found almost 10,000 kilometres away from Somerset on the Japanese island of Okinawa, which boasts so many centenarians among its population that the World Health Organization has dubbed it 'the island of long life'. Researchers looking for the causes of this happy state of affairs have ruled out some particular genetic advantage because people who have moved away to live elsewhere have not enjoyed the same longevity.

Okinawa has a mild climate and the population has good dietary habits, but it is now generally agreed that those factors are less important in accounting for their unusual degree of longevity than the cultural values of the people and the well-developed social life through which they celebrate and practise them. The way of life in Okinawa is characterized by a shared spiritual consciousness grounded in prayer, meditation, mindfulness and a determination to remain positive even in the face of adversity. The presiding value is *yuimahru* – the spirit of mutual co-operation, which is deeply rooted in the island's culture of lively group activity. It gives life meaning and generates the vitality which rings through the song they sing together each morning: 'The warmth of your heart prevents your body from rusting.' One imagines that they must also have a lot of fun. In contrast with most modern societies where too many of the old are afraid of becoming a nuisance and a burden, the people of Okinawa say, '*Tusui ya takara*', which means 'the elderly are our treasure'. In that respect, as in many others, their salutary way of life has a great deal to teach us.

From the moment we are born, we begin to learn how to relate to other human beings through the immediately intimate act of making eye contact. The first thing that babies recognize is their mother's eyes. As we grow and develop, through our innate skill at reading each other's facial expressions along with vocal tone and accompanying body language, we build and mature our relationships. Through those subtle forms of communication, acquired pre-verbally, an enormous amount of information is wordlessly exchanged. Face-to-face interaction shows us how people respond to the things we say and do. It's the medium through which we form and confirm friendships. As the poets have long insisted, it's through the eyes that we first fall in love, and because the ability to read each other's faces also alerts us to signs of immediate danger, it can effectively keep us alive.

Of course, it takes us years to fully develop the skills we need to be able to socialize successfully in a complex world, but those skills begin in infancy and childhood and the healthy development of social literacy will, to a large extent, be determined by how much time children are allowed to spend in face-to-face creative play and other intimate interactions with adults and other children. Fruitful communication depends on our ability to understand the emotional impact of our actions on those around us. Only through such understanding can we begin to move beyond a naïve self-centredness into fuller, more mature relationships. That way we eventually learn how to be good company. That way we come to recognize the life-promoting social value of compassion.

The work of Julianne Holt-Lunstad's team has graphically identified good social relationships as a marker of the chances of increased longevity. More widely, Susan Pinker's book emphasizes the therapeutic value of face-to-face social interaction in its insistence that 'neglecting to keep in close contact with people who are important to you is at least as dangerous to your health as a pack-a-day cigarette habit, hypertension, or obesity'. But to understand more completely the health-enhancing nature of strong personal connections, we also need to consider what is happening inside us, through the unconscious metabolic operations of the human body that take place, actively and responsively, as we engage in lively social interactions.

A BIOLOGICAL IMPERATIVE FOR COMPASSION

The importance of oxytocin was first identified by Henry Dale in 1906. This peptide hormone released by the pituitary gland plays an important role in childbirth by causing uterine contractions, so it was given a name derived from two Greek roots meaning 'sudden delivery'. Oxytocin also stimulates the flow of milk in the breast, thus assisting emotional bonding between mother and child. But later researchers have found that the release of oxytocin also has far wider effects that play a crucial role in many other important aspects of human life and behaviour.

At the immediately physical level, this versatile hormone has a role to play in the healing of wounds and acts as an anti-inflammatory. At the emotional level it eases depression and is associated with increased relaxation and feelings of trust. More famously, it also plays a significant part in the subtle processes of bonding between adults and is so deeply implicated in sexual attraction and erotic activity that it has commonly come to be known as 'the love hormone'. Normally functioning human beings love to love, and love to be loved, and the release of this hormone, which also acts as a neurotransmitter, plays such a vital role in the mediation of those rewarding emotions that in many ways we might be said to be oxytocin junkies.

Continuing research into the attributes of this ubiquitous hormone is revealing still more physiological and behavioural effects which contribute to our long-term bodily and psychological health. For present purposes, however, it's enough to emphasize that its release is stimulated by good social relationships. We can feel its presence and effects even during such brief episodes of social contact as chatting positively with someone who we have casually bumped into in the street.

As an example of how important such apparently light exchanges can be, a well-known journalist told one of the authors of this book how the thing he had missed most while he was embedded with a tight crew of war correspondents in Afghanistan was the kind of easy social contact that happened back home when chatting with other parents as they watched their children playing sport. In Frome, as we shall explore in the next chapter, it has been the development of easy places where people can come and just have a casual chat that has played such a crucial part in bringing back the heart into the town, and for some individuals it feels like this has literally saved their life.

An unconscious element in the satisfaction derived from those and similar occasions is the series of short bursts of oxytocin released by such relaxed interaction. But rather than thinking of the experience reductively as a merely hormonal event, it can be better understood as a feedback loop between active social behaviour and a subtle bodily function, which is mediated by and through hormones. We can recognize the value and importance of such moments consciously as they unfold, but our unconscious hormonal response helps the process along and the strengthening of those patterns of behaviour through physiological and biochemical changes further assists the development and maturing of good social literacy. In other words, compassion leads to connection which makes us feel good. Oxytocin is opposite in its function to the stress pathways which are also built into our metabolism. We all know that prolonged emotional tension and irascible responses are likely to be detrimental to good relationships, but they can also damage us physically by increasing blood pressure to harmful levels and by stimulating biochemical, pro-inflammatory pathways. These stress pathways will help to protect us from harm in the short term but, no matter what the cause, the activation of long-term stress responses will significantly weaken our health in many ways. That is a good recipe for the kind of chronic disease which eventually crowds doctors' surgeries and hospital wards.

To make matters worse, we may attempt to deal with the emotional consequences of stress in a variety of unhelpful ways, including resort to various addictions – comfort food, alcohol or drugs – which put our well-being further at risk. Once that happens, it's easy to get caught in a vicious circle of declining health aggravated by increasing stress. But the medical evidence is now clearly established: we can improve our health and well-being through successful relationships subtly mediated by hormonal response and other biological processes and we can avoid the harmful impacts of stress through the care and development of those same social relationships. In both contexts, compassion lies at the heart of the matter.

At the most basic level of our own existence, such hormones facilitate the act of procreation which has allowed our species to survive and flourish. But they also foster bonding at the more mature emotional levels of friendship and love. We find biochemical and hormonal messengers busily at work in creating efficient social relationships wherever we look, and it has become clear that, from an evolutionary perspective, we cannot separate our behaviour from our biochemistry. Crucial to both is that capacity for compassion on which social survival ultimately depends.

IT TAKES A COMMUNITY FOR AN INDIVIDUAL TO THRIVE

An overly simple, sometimes ideologically driven, reading of Darwin has emphasized the power of competition as the dominant evolutionary force – 'the survival of the fittest', as Herbert Spencer defined it, in a world red in tooth and claw. But such a view underestimates the vital role of co-operation as a complementary force without which life would be intolerable and survival improbable. Like most other species, human beings are social animals, and at a deep biological level we understand that compassion is the essential bonding agent of good social relationships. But while the same hormones may be found in humans and animals, the hormonal release associated with our feelings of compassion is more than a random product of evolution. Biochemistry is not a chance evolutionary act moving in a random direction: rather, it is a process of refinement which has been happening over hundreds of millions of years. So perhaps a more appropriate phrase than survival of the fittest is survival of the most compassionate.

Because compassion is so deeply embedded inside us, we can all recognize moments when those feelings motivate us to act to reduce suffering in others. It might be an act as simple as a mother feeding her baby after hearing the child cry or helping an anxious old person to cross a busy street. Such moments happen repeatedly throughout our lives and we are able to respond in this way because the aptitude for compassion is inherent within us – a precious resource that, if properly developed, can be applied in all our social interactions wherever we go.

From our earliest days as hunters and gatherers, we have always known that, in most of our activities, we can achieve more by working as a group than we can as solitary individuals. Even in a highly mobile, industrialized society which now mostly consists of nuclear families, bringing up children is a group activity and life feels easier and more pleasurable when we get help from family or friends with what can sometimes be a burdensome duty. More importantly, knowledge of how best to rear children is passed down across generations and, for that reason, grandparents still have an important role to play, both with their own grandchildren and with others in their neighbourhood. But we live in times when increased social mobility has severely disrupted the patterns of extended family life. Much may have been gained through that change, but much has also been lost, and the severing of easy, frequent contact across the generations of family life is among the more poignant of such losses. To that and wider processes of sociological change, which now include increased divorce statistics, must be added those pressures of technological change which widen the cultural gap between generations with deranging velocity. Today's grandchildren, accustomed as they are to fast-speed visual stimulation, may find it hard to relate to their grandparents' stories and advice. But if such generational links break down, the quality of childcare is likely to deteriorate, so the patience and concerned interest shown to the young by their caring grandparents is, as the people of Okinawa insist, a priceless resource. In much the same way, it's also increasingly clear that children educated in schools where teachers pay proper attention to the personal welfare and social cohesion of the pupils are more likely to develop the essential skills of social literacy.

The beneficial value of good social relations also becomes evident when we ourselves, or someone close to us, falls ill. Their support amounts to more than a matter of offering the warmth of sympathetic friendship. Problem solving is often done much better by a team of willing helpers than by an individual acting alone. Their collective knowledge can direct the person in need towards more effective treatment strategies and help them to identify the best mode of medical intervention. In more immediately practical terms, group assistance with shopping, cooking and cleaning, accompanied by expressions of affection, laughter and friendship, can transform a situation where a solitary carer may be putting his or her own health at risk into a shared experience which, even amidst the sadness of grief, loss and bereavement, can prove life enhancing for all.

A CHOICE BETWEEN COMPETITION AND COMPASSION

As humans, we swim in a sea of compassion. We feel its effects at work in the biochemistry of our hormones, in our individual physiology and in our patterns of behaviour as we function together well in social groups. But if we think of compassion merely as a pleasant way to relate that we may occasionally practise in the course of our lives, we are missing the point! Whether we know it or not, it is built into the very fabric of our bodies. It is present daily when we simply ask a friend how they are faring or make them a welcome cup of tea. And it is essential to our social functioning because we are interdependent beings ultimately reliant on the quiet presence of compassion for our survival.

That said, some readers may feel that, in its eagerness to emphasize the role of compassion, this chapter has paid scant attention to the countervailing fact that the aggressive force of competition, and the urge for dominance within hierarchical systems, may also, for sound evolutionary reasons, be hard-wired into our nature and behaviour. Rather than examining in detail an issue which is manifestly evident both in the animal world and in so much of what happens every day in the contentious arena of human affairs, the aim here has been to achieve a necessary rebalancing of perspective on the issue. The need for such rebalancing becomes increasingly evident and urgent as a drastic lack of balance in that respect now endangers the continuing life of many species including our own. At the same time, it would be naïve to underestimate the difficulties of translating feelings of compassion into effectively transformative action in what is a fiercely competitive world. Such a process of change demands both imaginative vision and resolute courage. But that things can be done to achieve it is evidenced by the remarkable success of the Compassionate Frome project.

Through a detailed study of what has been happening there, the next chapter will describe in more detail what has been happening in Frome and examine ways in which the transforming power of compassion can be effectively activated, both in individuals and in communities. It will show how by harnessing that power to the inter-relationship of health and social welfare, a healthcare service which is affordable in its costs and more comprehensive in its effects can be integrated within the wider pattern of community life.

Once we fully acknowledge the role of compassion in our lives and begin to take advantage of the rich resources it puts at our disposal, we can improve both our health and happiness. Its benevolent power can even keep us alive for longer and reduce our chances of ending our days in a hospital ward. It can also, when imaginatively applied, revitalize the life of whole communities.

That such a vision is more than an abstract, ideologically constructed strategy which may sound good on paper but bears little relationship to matters on the ground, will become apparent in the very human stories that the success of the Compassionate Frome project has to tell.

CHAPTER 5

COMPASSION IN ACTION

Never doubt that a small group of thoughtful, committed citizens
can change the world; indeed, it's the only thing that ever has.

Margaret Mead

T he decades since Margaret Thatcher, in an interview for
Woman's Own in 1987, notoriously declared that 'There is
no such thing as society' have witnessed a radical shift in the
value system underpinning the political and economic management
of human affairs. That shift has been far-ranging in its effects on the
lives of both individuals and communities. Its underlying principle
has been accurately summarized by the distinguished psychoanalyst
David Bell, director of the Fitzjohn's Unit of the Tavistock and
Portman NHS Foundation Trust. In his introduction to the book
Against the Tide, Bell writes, 'Neoliberalism, which manifests itself
as the increasing penetration of the market form into all spheres
of life, including healthcare, has led to the near hegemony of a
world-view in which society is (mis)understood as an aggregate of
individuals, each seeking to satisfy his or her own needs.'

Bell claims that, in the field of psychiatry, the consequence of
this shift has been an 'industrialization of human suffering', in

which the tendency is to view the patient as 'a passive recipient of a pathological process' – that is, as an example of one or more of a number of well-categorized mental illnesses – and who is therefore seen as an object of this process, not a subject. What gets lost from such an impersonal perspective, Bell insists, is a complex understanding of the individual as 'a unique being whose suffering occurs within the narrative of his or her lived life and the human relationships that surround him or her.' At the immediate level, those relationships will be personal and familial, but they are also societal, and the prevailing narrative determining the quality of life within the wider community will also have a direct and often oppressive bearing on the condition of the person suffering from mental distress. Fortunately, the results from the Compassionate Frome project also show how community life may have a transformative effect on individuals in any number of positive ways.

If Bell's diagnosis of the wider, impersonal forces affecting the quality of our social life is correct (and this book argues that it is), then it is not only the essentially personal value of the suffering individual's subjective identity that gets lost, but also an authentic sense of the true value of what the idea of community might mean. Or, to put it another way, the privatization and commodification of fundamental aspects of our lives by neoliberal market forces is inimical not only to the mental health of individuals but also to the health and vitality of the communities in which they live.

As society becomes ever more complex and fragmented, technocratic 'solutions' to the ensuing problems are designed by experts in various professionally defined fields and then imposed, top-down, as targeted schemes by politicians who are increasingly seen as out of touch with the lives of the people. (Politicians who, often enough, for example, govern the administration and curriculum of schools which their children do not attend and the organization and methods of public health and welfare systems which they do not use.)

As Bell insists, this neoliberal perspective on human affairs now dominates mainstream political and economic thinking worldwide. In virtually all areas of life, the centralized power of public decision-making is delegated to, or seized and controlled by those who aggressively seek it, along with the professional expertise of those technocrats who serve them. The consequence is a more or less intentionally promoted lack of trust in local communities to evaluate and understand their own immediate experience or to exercise appropriate control over their own affairs and way of life. Hence the sense of impotence felt by many individuals in the face of such impersonal forces and the growing discontent and mistrust that it generates.

The philosophy and practice of compassionate community development turns that increasingly unsatisfactory method of managing human affairs on its head. It does so by working from two assumptions which differ radically from those on which centralized authority is based:

1. That individuals have the capacity to define and solve their own problems.
2. That the communities in which they come together are rich in social assets, skills and talents.

These were the assumptions that underpinned the Compassionate Frome project from the start.

Its formal name within the NHS structure is Health Connections Mendip and its mission statement begins as follows:

Started in 2013, Health Connections Mendip has worked in an innovative, dynamic, organic way to create a model which is based on trust and doing what is right for/with people and the community. We look for opportunities and work alongside people to shine a light on the things that people want more of and want to share; and to help draw energy and creativity into areas where people want to get involved in finding their own solutions to things that are important to them. By being the glue and helping create connections we have shown the impact of a can-do model that is based on trust, kindness, creativity and connections.

The replicable success of the Frome model has demonstrated that such an approach is capable of improving the health and welfare of individuals by reducing the rate of emergency admissions to hospitals, while at the same time enhancing the general vitality of community life. Those remarkable results were achieved by three key measures.

- Firstly, the social resources already available in the town were identified and collated – those clubs, choirs, charities and societies already bringing people together in shared activities that incidentally generate the warmth, conviviality, laughter and friendship that are core characteristics of a compassionate community.
- Next, appropriate support was given to maximize the potential of these resources through appropriate publicity and backing.
- Then, previously unidentified needs were recognized and imaginative means to meet them put in place by drawing on local skills and talents, along with such professional expertise and funding as might be deemed helpful to turn those gaps into opportunities for further creative development.

In this way, the situation of individuals suffering from various incapacitating illnesses and social isolation of the kind which can, if left unattended, lead to desperation and suicide, were brought into the embrace of a widening network of friendship and support.

Together, Dr Helen Kingston and Jenny Hartnoll instigated a programme of change by focusing in practical terms on what was needed, what was possible and what made sense.

TRUSTING THE COMMUNITY

In some respects, Jenny Hartnoll brought an unconventional background to the work. Not having the confidence to believe that she would succeed either at art school or in academia, she dropped out of university. As a result of this decision, she eventually came to the realization that her principal strength lay in the kind of creativity that makes things happen. After travelling abroad and training as a dance and movement therapist, she worked in a number of areas, including helping those with drug and alcohol addiction, learning disabilities or suffering from mental health problems.

Eventually she set up her own charity, renting space in the depressed London district of Harlesden where people from a poor, largely immigrant community could come together to exchange goods and join in social events. That space performed a function that was once the role of the high street – a place where people created and sustained social relationships while shopping for the necessities of life in a way that now rarely happens along the aisles of supermarkets. The activities that attracted people into that space held their own interest, but the principal benefits accrued from that incidental magic through which spirits are lifted, mutual support and encouragement are given and new friendships formed.

So, with irrepressible enthusiasm, Jenny persuaded Next and other companies to donate children's clothes to her charity and Dorling Kindersley to donate unsold books. She ran dance and movement classes for parents and their children and supported the organization of other events which brought people together around a variety of interests and activities.

'We worked with the whole community in Brent,' she says of that time. 'It was amazing to see people learning English through singing songs together. I had someone come up to me who said, "You didn't know at the time, but I had post-natal depression. Coming to your group was the thing that saved me." There were so many of those kinds of stories.'

Through such affirmative experiences the seeds of what would eventually become Health Connections Mendip were first sown in her imagination.

However, when Jenny and her family moved from London to Frome, she was not immediately able to continue such deeply satisfying work. Instead she worked as a health coach for a community partnership in an NHS project that hoped to reduce emergency admissions to hospital by supporting individuals at risk in their efforts to live healthier lives.

Earlier NHS programmes designed to deal more aggressively and proactively with chronic disease had directed GPs to manage the care of people seriously at risk of hospitalization through greater attention to medical detail and to convince patients to undertake programmes of improved self-management. But it soon became clear that to over-medicalize the condition of people suffering from chronic disease only exacerbates the need for more medical services.

When neither of these approaches succeeded in reducing hospital admissions, a new initiative – that of health coaching – was introduced. Its underlying assumption was that, by and large, people are too incompetent to manage their own illness and therefore need to be coached in better practice by an expert guide. Though this may sound like an efficient approach, its effect is to identify the illness as the subject and the patient as the object, in much the same way that David Bell diagnosed the inadequacy of much psychiatric treatment. In a wider context, it also fails to answer a problem with which most GPs are depressingly familiar – that of the increasing number of people presenting at their surgeries whose principal cause of suffering is the loneliness caused by social isolation.

GETTING TO THE COMPASSIONATE ROOT OF ILLNESS

To understand the relationship between social isolation and severe illness more clearly, one might consider the case of an isolated elderly person suffering from diabetes. This chronic disease is caused by high levels of insulin resulting from excessive exposure to sugars. Left unattended, high blood sugar levels will eventually cause serious damage to multiple bodily organs. The dangers of the disease can be managed through improved diet and exercise along with appropriate medication, but if the patient is also desperately lonely the motivation provided by a well-intentioned health coach to sustain such efforts may not be sufficient to improve the situation. The patient may even collude with the disease to put an end to their misery. However, if that underlying problem is addressed by giving the patient opportunities to discover the kind of supportive companionship that new friendships can give then the chances are good that a renewed sense of having something to live for will increase their desire to take better care of themselves, to regain their mobility and to get out into the world.

Jenny Hartnoll had learned from her experience in London that the act of bringing people together in convivial circumstances could have a powerful impact on their general well-being. So, even while working in the relatively limited role of a health trainer, she began to assemble information about social resources already active in Frome and the surrounding area. The website she developed helped to make this information conveniently available both to herself and to others, but when she asked her employers for backing to develop her ideas for harnessing those resources to a socially-based programme of healthcare, she was promptly told it would take too much time and cost too much money.

Reflecting on that period in her life, Jenny says, 'Obvious things needed to be done, but my hands were tied and I wasn't allowed to do the job. So I did it in my own time because I don't necessarily see those boundaries. If someone at work tells me I can't do something, I don't think, "I can't do that." I think, "I'm a human being, of course I can do that."'

And there we have it: the essential first step in harnessing the power of compassion is to see what needs to be done and then to get on and do it. Determination sometimes requires defiance and Jenny was not deterred by the refusal of management to give her the go-ahead to act in response to what she saw as an obvious need. The nature and role of management as an aid or an obstacle to positive action is a theme which will be considered later but, for the moment, it's enough to say that Jenny's determination clearly demonstrated that people who actually do the work are the best judges of what is needed to make things run more efficiently. The authority of managers rests on positions of seniority which may put them out of touch with coal-face realities and restrict their thinking. Recognizing this brings to light a fundamental principle for bringing about creative and compassionate change.

PARTICIPATORY COMMUNITY DEVELOPMENT

The insights arising from Jenny Hartnoll's experience in Harlesden had led her to the belief that the simple act of bringing people together in lively social relationship could help them to recognize and define their own problems and then work their way towards appropriate solutions. Beyond those immediately pragmatic considerations many other benefits would accrue simply as an unplanned by-product of increased communication and convivial activity.

The success of her previous work in those respects demonstrated a wider social parallel to the kind of problem she encountered with management in her professional work as a health trainer. More widely, it points to the difference between two contrasting approaches to community development.

The first, most commonly applied approach is based on official strategies devised by expert professionals appointed by people in authority who tend to work by defining deficiencies and coming up with rational plans for their solution. The other approach is based in the community's knowledge and experience of its own strengths, skills and resources, and relies on its capacity to come up with organic, bespoke responses to its own needs and problems, while calling on professional expertise where its advice is clearly essential. This latter approach is fundamental to the emergence of a truly participatory process of community development.

That process begins with the communities themselves. In initiatives such as co-production or co-development the assumption is sometimes that communities are junior partners whose acquiescence in schemes determined by experts can largely be taken for granted. The professionals decide that there is a problem in need of solution and then institute a consultation process with the people affected by the problem to seek views on how it might be solved.

But participatory development goes further than that. Through their associational life gathered together within the community, the people themselves define and establish the priorities for action.

Jenny has used this way of working right from the beginning. Whilst mapping all the wide-ranging groups in the community, she was aware that it was not all inclusive and gaps were present. Part of the way of working for Health Connections Mendip has been to wait for suggestions to arise from the community and then support people in turning these suggestions into action. For example, someone who suffered from multiple sclerosis wanted to meet other people who also had this disease. Jenny and her team helped her organise a local group. Likewise, someone from the sixth form college wanted to become a community connector. Jenny helped her set up a patient participation group at the college, making it the youngest group in the country. The advice of experts and professionals may be sought as necessary, but it is not a prerequisite of the whole process.

A great example of effective community-minded action that came about almost organically, answering a need felt by many and bringing them together for the benefit of all, is Parkrun. Parkrun was started by Paul Sinton-Hewitt in 2004. Paul had been training for the London marathon, but an injury meant he was no longer able to run with his usual club. He had also recently lost his job and was worried about feeling isolated. He invited some friends to run five kilometres with him in London's Bushy Park and then they all went for coffee afterwards.

There are now Parkruns in 20 countries around the world, in locations as far apart as Moscow, Walvis Bay, Namibia and Tokyo. It's estimated that three million people have taken part in a Parkrun. The events are completely free and open to everyone, including beginners, the overweight, the elderly, wheelchair users, people pushing prams and club runners alike. You can try to run a personal best or jog round as slowly as you like. Everyone can simply turn up and not be judged, just accepted for who they are. This compassionate approach is surely at the heart of the project's overwhelming success.

We are continuously told we should exercise more but if the motivation is not there to do it, we will not go. However, if going for a run means spending time with friends, maybe even meeting some strangers for a chat, then getting out and doing it becomes a lot easier. Creating the right environment for these important components is the essential feature of its success.

These important elements are almost a blueprint of how and what we should be thinking about when designing group activities. Looking at the strengths of this simple community-minded action, it fulfils the function of supportive social relationships. The original Parkrun ended by participants going somewhere for a cup of coffee. It meant from the beginning there was time to chat and develop friendships. The running is an excuse for the important bit, which is the social relationships, the love, laughter and friendship, that happen along the way.

THE SERVICE DIRECTORY

Given that communities already deploy many rich resources to benefit the lives of their members, the first sensible step in creating a compassionate health-related programme of social development is to map the full range of these resources and make the information widely available to the community in a directory of available services.

Drawing such a map and compiling a directory raises the question of what actually constitutes a community resource. At the simplest level, it can be defined as anywhere that people are free to gather together. Beyond that, the key characteristic for current purposes is that it is a place where people can feel confident to establish and strengthen relationships and friendships, often through sharing common interests. That said, it is necessary to stress that compassion – a genuine care for the welfare of others – should be an active, even if unspoken, value behind such gatherings. For a variety of reasons, people sometimes gather for harmful purposes. A compassionate community will flourish by building and supporting those gatherings which have benevolent intentions.

A wide variety of leisure activities fall under that general heading, including interests as diverse as sports clubs, walking groups, horticulture, country dancing, knit-and-chat groups, reading circles, weaving workshops and choirs, along with many other hobbies and preoccupations around which people spontaneously gather.

The directory will also include information about groups in which the members are directly engaged with specific health and social care issues, such as those suffering from the same disease or disability or struggling with related challenges of loneliness and isolation. Existing voluntary agencies and services dealing with such matters as bereavement counselling, housing or transport problems, and matters of general guidance and advice, will also feature on the service directory. The design of the directory is as important as its content and for Jenny the key was that it should be easy to use. Given a budget to build the directory, Jenny recruited help with its design but, as is often the case with IT projects, the process became frustratingly long and arduous. Knowing what she wanted and having a good idea how she would use it, one weekend she set to and came up with a design of her own. That same design is still in use four years later.

At this point it may be helpful to take a look at the service directory for Health Connections Mendip as an example of a website that has been tried and tested through extensive use by both the professionals and the community it serves. It can be found by searching 'directory Health Connections Mendip', or at www.healthconnectionsmendip.org/mendip-directory.

The directory is accessed through a single click on the Health Connections Mendip website. A brief introductory note reads:

> Do you want to find groups and services in the community that might help improve your health and wellbeing?
>
> Do you live in Mendip, Somerset? Do you have a long-term health condition? Would you like support in developing your knowledge, skills and confidence in order to help you better manage your long-term health conditions?
>
> If the answer to the above is yes, then have a look at all the support that is available in Mendip by using our Directory of Services or book an appointment for one to one support with a Health Connector.

The page lists about 50 items of group help and support as broad categories. This list has been developed pragmatically, simply by knowing which categories were being used the most, and contains general items – such as bereavement, exercise, well-being and smoking – along with more specific ones referring to information and groups concerned with particular conditions such as Parkinson's disease, multiple sclerosis or dementia.

Clicking on a category reveals a further list of individual items. Each item has some information about its subject, together with contact details and group meeting times. The site makes it easy to save the items to a basket for later printing or to print them individually. The simple form in which the information is provided means that vital details are immediately available without trawling through the text. If areas of interest or concern arise spontaneously in conversation between doctor and patient, it is easy to drill down to find something that might be worth investigating further.

For example, clicking on the bereavement link reveals a list of 30 items, ranging from sources of counselling for those suffering from the death of a child, or of a much-loved pet, to the Frome Coffee and Cake Bereavement Support Group. The diversity of themes and concerns gathered under each general category makes it simple to home in on whatever offers of information, help, advice, encouragement and support feel most relevant to individual circumstances.

To ensure its current usefulness, the directory is constantly kept updated by the Health Connections Mendip team. If a group closes down or changes the time when it meets, that information can be immediately subtracted or added by one of the team without any need to relay it to a separate IT department to be acted on at some indeterminate point later.

TALKING CAFÉS

However necessary and useful the directory would prove, Jenny knew from the outset that it would not be sufficient in itself to create vital links between individuals and the community. After all, not everyone is happy using the internet and elderly people in particular might find it uncongenial to seek out information they need by using a website. And so, in 2013, Health Connections Mendip set up the first talking café to be established in the UK.

Jenny tells the story of the informal way in which that came about:

There were people coming to me saying I don't want a specific support group, I just want to meet other people. So I thought that 'a talking café' sounded a nice title. I put it in the diary – if I put something in the diary, I know it will always happen. The first one was held in the Cheese and Grain in Frome. The place wasn't usually open on a Monday morning but they agreed to open the café really early. There were no groups using the space upstairs so I invited in the Health Walks group and helped to set up meetings for the MS exercise group. People were soon streaming into what had been an empty space to do these exercise groups. It built up an energy down there. Then a job club started upstairs.

The talking café is simply a place where people are free to meet informally and talk about anything that matters to them. There are no membership rules, no agendas that determine the topics of conversation and new people are always warmly welcomed. The invitation is simple and in the name, and the reason people turn up is to talk, often just wanting to chat with others who feel the same way. In defiance of the stereotype of formal stiffness long-associated with British people, the success of the Frome talking cafés demonstrates that, when given the opportunity, people are more than ready and willing to engage in conversation with people they have never previously met. They do it in ways which may simply be a pleasurable means of passing a morning or may be the start of a rich new pattern of friendship. Taking part in such a relaxed social arrangement can even change lives. As Barbara touchingly put it, 'If it wasn't for the talking café I would have a lonely experience. It has helped me look forward to getting up on Monday morning.' There are now several such cafés meeting regularly in a number of venues across Frome and more widely in the surrounding area. At every talking café someone from Health Connections Mendip, or a trained community connector, will be present in case people are in need of specific information or want to be signposted to a place where they are able to find things out for themselves.

Joe was 92 years old when he first visited the talking café. On retiring from the army, he had become a butcher and then ran a grocery in Staffordshire. After the death of his first wife, he remarried and went to live in Wales and then subsequently moved to Blackpool where, within a short space of time, his wife suffered a brain haemorrhage and was left permanently disabled. Now a full-time carer for his wife, Joe had recently moved to Frome to be closer to his daughter. Recently, he too had suffered a stroke and had come down to the talking café to get to know people. 'With having to look after my wife, I can't get out and have not been anywhere. It's good to talk to people. I don't get a chance to socialize otherwise.'

Through attending the talking café and participating in conversations that spontaneously arise there, people are able to make connections with other group activities in the town. Having lived in Wells after his retirement, Patrick Abrahams moved to Frome because of the friendly nature of the town and started the Men's Shed there. Men's Shed is a nationwide movement in which men, and women for Women's Sheds, can meet together and take part in a common interest of making and mending. As with other groups, the common interest is a way of people coming together, with the by-product of love, laughter and friendship. It is the social connectedness that makes it so powerful, in marked contrast to spending solitary time alone in a shed. The Men's Shed association supports the running of groups across the UK.

A regular attender at the talking café, Patrick Abrahams says:

I love coming down here, meeting all kinds of people. You can meet someone who has just arrived and may be isolated and lonely. It can be hard for people to go through the door into a new room full of people. I can invite them to the Shed and they will say, 'Will you be there?'. They need to know when they go through the door that they can say 'hi' to someone they know. It's really beneficial to allow people to join softly without any commitment. They will often see people who are like them, be it man or woman, young or old.

On his local radio show *Shed Happens* on Frome FM, Patrick interviewed Matt, who described how he had come to join the Men's Shed when he was off work, following an intense period of stress:

I had a bit of a breakdown at work. I was diagnosed with depression. The doctor suggested I go down the Cheese and Grain to have a chat with people. That appealed to me. I thought the depression was all my fault. But you are not judged at the talking café or the shed. I met up with Patrick who suggested I came along to the Men's Shed. I met the most amazing guys I think I have ever met. Had a chat, no one was there to judge and there were other people who had problems similar to myself. I came down to the shed for four months. I developed the confidence in myself I needed to go back to work. If it wasn't for the shed I don't know where I would be. The confidence the guys gave me – advice, just chatting and not judging. I realized it was my work that had put me into depression. All along I thought it was me, it was my fault, but coming down the shed turned things around.

The Women's Shed in Frome has a similar convivial purpose. One woman had been suffering long months of lonely bereavement following the death of her husband; she was told about a place where women were gathering socially to chat together as they made various items that could be sold by local charities. She had no idea that the Women's Shed had been formed as part of a wider community project, which was exactly as it should be – when she decided to go along it felt like a natural occurrence in her life, meeting an essential need, that had happened spontaneously as a result of a friendly, informal conversation. She found that she was warmly welcomed by a group of women, some of whom had only recently come to Frome and were looking to make new friends. Her spirit was lifted and the whole feel of her life changed by joining the group.

COMMUNITY CONNECTORS

Though much thought, care and planning went into the creation of the Health Connections Mendip project, the course of its subsequent development has largely been determined through imaginative responses to perceived local needs. Where gaps in the provision of local services appeared, and a routine medical approach alone was an insufficient response, new social capital was built by drawing on the knowledge, skills and resources of members of the community to come up with appropriate solutions. There was no five-year plan or complicated document setting out its development.

Jenny Hartnoll had seen how people's well-being could be improved by connecting them to peer support groups or appropriate social agencies. Community health champions – a voluntary position – can be key agents in this. They are defined by the National Health Service as:

People who, with training and support, bring their ability to relate to people and their own life experience to transform health and well-being in their communities. Within their families, communities and

*workplaces they empower and motivate people to get involved in
healthy social activities, create groups to meet local needs and signpost
people to relevant support and services. They also help others to enjoy
healthier lives by raising awareness of health and healthy choices,
sharing health messages, removing barriers and creating supportive
networks and environments.*

Jenny knew that the work of such people would be an immensely
beneficial asset to the work of Health Connections Mendip, but the
intensive training programme for a health champion takes up to
nine hours, which seemed an unrealistic expectation to impose on
local volunteers, so she devised a briefer, two-hour period of training
to suit local needs, to create a team of local 'community connectors'.
The programme would first explain the way the project fitted into
the provision of healthcare and social welfare and then show how
the directory of local resources could be used by the community
connectors to bring help and support to those in need. The training
began on a small scale but, as news began to spread, interest grew
and more people turned up for training until quite soon a team of
over one thousand community connectors was active throughout
Frome and the surrounding area.

Though the title 'community connector' may have a slightly
official ring, it simply describes human beings who have become
socially efficient at deploying their own good nature, whether as
a friend, neighbour or casual acquaintance. The range of people
trained as community connectors around Frome is now remarkably
wide. They are beacons of compassion in the community. Simply
by having information at their fingertips, their natural compassion
comes into play whenever called upon as they go about their lives.

The principle on which their work is based is very simple. It
draws on that deep well of compassion that makes its otherwise

unrecognized presence clearly felt when, in the normal course of conversation, we hear about another person's troubles and feel a natural desire to help. The problem is that we don't always know what the best way of helping might be. The motivation may be there, but without adequate means to put it into action we are at a loss. However, if we have access to a directory of local resources and are trained in its use, we are equipped to become more than a sympathetic bystander. We know where appropriate help can be found and how to share or 'signpost' someone to that knowledge. What might have been only a kindly conversation now has somewhere to go.

A quietly expressed need for help, support or advice can arise spontaneously in many different contexts – while chatting to one's hairdresser, for example, or overhearing by chance someone talking in a pub. A person clearly in distress after a recent bereavement might be helped by the knowledge that a group of such people meets for mutual support and consolation at the health centre or in a talking café every other week. Information about similar meetings for carers might come as a blessing to a person exhausted by the demands of coping alone with a partner suffering from dementia. The larger the number of trained connectors who are active in a community, the more likely it becomes that such helpful conversations will happen and the greater the impact on the overall quality of community life.

In addition to hairdressers, bartenders and café proprietors, trained community connectors include, among others, taxi drivers, shopkeepers, pharmacists, police community support workers and school sixth-formers. Professionals such as police officers, ambulance paramedics and accident and emergency staff who meet people in all kinds of trouble can also make good use of a trained knowledge of community resources to direct people to the help they may urgently need. It is, in fact, a role open to anyone who wishes to train.

Lotte, who runs a café in Frome, has been trained as a community connector. Describing what it means, she says, 'It is being aware of and being available to people. We are just connecting people really. We can direct them to websites, phone numbers or groups. People are compassionate in Frome. They like to feel they are part of something.'

Frome's community connector training programme is run by Julie Carey-Downes, who originally qualified as a psychiatric nurse and went on to train as a lawyer. Neither of these jobs greatly attracted her, so she applied for the position when she saw it advertised in the local press, was appointed and became so involved in the whole project that she subsequently became a health connector too. In talking about her job satisfaction, Julie describes how the community police officers who joined the programme reported afterwards that the community connector training was the most useful they had ever received. She explains:

> They felt that during their working life, they now actually had somewhere they could signpost people to when they were struggling with life's hard circumstances. In addition, they have made direct referrals to health connectors as part of their role as community police officers. Other people trained as community connectors report back that they never knew there was so much out there in the community.

Significantly, many people whose first contact with the project was prompted by the pressing needs of their personal situation have since trained to become community connectors themselves.

A year after the training programme had begun, Jenny sent out a questionnaire to the team of connectors active in and around Frome asking how often they had held conversations linking people to community resources, either through the web directory or the talking cafés, or simply supplying them with the phone number of Health Connections Mendip. Half of them replied and, on average, they claimed to have had about 20 conversations a year. Since then, a steady flow of people has passed through the programme until, after four years, over a thousand people have been trained. This means that, among a population of around a hundred thousand residents in the Mendip district of Somerset, possibly somewhere around twenty thousand conversations linking people to the various resources listed in the directory happen every year.

Simply by relying on the goodwill and compassion of ordinary people, and by providing them with the tools to access good information, Jenny Hartnoll and her team at Health Connections Mendip have made it possible for almost everyone in the local community to be reached in time of need by simple word of mouth.

HEALTH CONNECTORS

As a natural consequence of people coming to her for advice, Jenny found herself engaged in a considerable amount of one-to-one work. Eventually the demands these meetings made on her time became so overwhelming that they restricted her ability to concentrate on the community development aspect of her job. If she was to build and support the range of community resources she envisioned, other people would have to take over some of the one-to-one work. The need for this additional assistance led her to introduce the role of health connectors to the programme.

Health connectors are not healthcare professionals. They are people who, among other things, have been trained in the techniques of motivational interviewing that grew out of clinical psychology. Simply put, this is a way of working with people to get them to formulate their goals as clearly as possible and then to take actions that will lead to the achievement of those goals.

The nature of the relationship between the health connector and the patient differs somewhat from that of the health professional. The health professional uses the consultation process to determine the cause of the presenting problem and then apply the treatment that should yield the best possible solution to that problem, whereas the role of the health connector is to focus on the patient's overall well-being.

Having an illness has an impact on the rest of life, and likewise life has an impact on how we experience illness. Simply addressing disease and symptoms will not always resolve either the problems that may have created the illness in the first place or life's difficulties that arise from falling ill.

Such issues will be considered in more detail later, but for now it's enough to note that the combination of good disease control with good symptom management and well-co-ordinated care do not necessarily equate to a good sense of well-being. If both health and well-being are the aim, then attention must be paid to both these areas. Furthermore, because they are not separate, they affect each other, so if we want to treat either, we will have to treat both.

The health connector's training in motivational interviewing equips them to find out through careful questioning what matters most to the person they are working with. Because each person is different, the health connector does not make assumptions about what that might be. The aim is to keep an open mind while listening to what the patient has to say about the problems with which they are struggling and then use that as the basis on which to work through them.

Consider again the situation of elderly diabetics. They are probably less mobile than they were, friends may have died and their ability to get out and socialize with new people can be limited. A crass, overly simplistic response to such a complaint would be to say, 'You need to get out more' – words which are commonly heard in many GP practices. A better way forward is to find out what form of social contact might be most meaningful. If the patient can get out of the house, the conversation with the health connector would explore the kind of activity that might engage their interest and give them pleasure. This might be simply chatting with other people or, more ambitiously, perhaps joining a choir. The solution is tailored to match their interests.

The patient may need a lift to get to the choir, or perhaps they would like the health connector to accompany them to the first meeting, giving them the confidence to walk through the door into a room full of strangers. Strangers are, of course, potential friends, but that can be hard to remember when feeling both shy and isolated. The offer of company could make the challenge more manageable. Alternatively, patients who can no longer get out of the house might welcome visits from a befriending volunteer.

Truly compassionate help treats people as equals and is both tactfully inquisitive and respectful. Any less considerate, or more self-assertive, response to a patient's situation is likely to deter them from taking any further part in constructive conversation.

In this crucial respect, the attitude and approach of the health connector is the same as that of a good community development worker. Both start from the belief that the people they serve are rich in resourcefulness. Though a measure of support may be needed to help them through the difficulties that confront them, both health connector and development worker understand that support is what is done *with* people rather than *to* them, and that the single valid assumption is that the necessary tools for improvement of a personal or community situation are already present and waiting to be used.

BUILDING COMMUNITY RESOURCES FROM THE GROUND UP

As health connectors go about their work visiting people across the community, their attention may be drawn to needs that remain as yet unmet. For example, in a village where there is no formally organized befriending service – be that a charitable organization or other volunteer group – available to a patient, the health connector might look for ways to enlist the help of the informal networks that already exist in a village where long-term residents already know each other well. Consultation between the health connector and a community development worker could lead to an appropriate strategy for developing a more widely available service. A piece in the parish magazine suggesting that a befriending service would be a blessing to the lonely people in the neighbourhood might prompt a meeting in the village hall. Someone present who already knows the people in need of care could then be given support to start a voluntary group. That way, the lonely would be served and the bonds of village life strengthened.

It might prove more difficult for health connectors to kickstart that kind of initiative in an urban environment, but an appropriate strategy could be to approach an existing church group or organized charity that might be interested in building a befriending service. Some hospices already run this kind of service. For example, St Joseph's Hospice in the London borough of Hackney runs a scheme called Compassionate Neighbours which builds and supports friendships across a multicultural community. The increased social cohesion that comes from the mixing of individuals from different ethnic groups during training sessions and the growth of friendly relationships and greater understanding among previously isolated people are some of the many benefits accruing from this kind of programme. Furthermore, as Jenny Hartnoll insists, the immediate impact of the programme on the lives of individuals has a ripple effect that passes on to influence the attitudes of families and friends who learn how someone they know is helping both themselves and others to live a richer life.

In Frome, talking cafés have been shown to be an effective community resource, acting as mini community hubs. For example, peer-support bereavement groups and disease-specific groups have been started through the cafés to help those suffering from, or caring for people with, such gravely disabling conditions as Parkinson's disease or dementia. These informal groups are a simple response to needs of individuals within the community and an alert community development worker will find means to give those groups the support they need. Sometimes there is a clear need for such a group but no one willing to set it up. For this reason, Health Connections Mendip stepped in and started to create group self-management programmes designed to help people with chronic health conditions to manage their disease. Social connectedness is vital to a person's well-being, but it's also essential that their illness – be it chronic lung disease, heart disease or diabetes – is carefully managed through proper attention to their medication regime and relevant aspects of their lifestyle. In Frome, a self-management programme might last for around six weeks, but Jenny and her team have discovered that many people who have benefited from membership of such a group want to build on the gains they have made and continue to sustain their friendships with people they first met in the group. Health Connections Mendip developed a second group following on from the self-management group, so that attendees could maintain both the physical gains they achieved as well as continue to meet with the friends they had made. These friendships deepen and have continued for many years.

THE WHOLE PICTURE

The term Community *Development Service* is somewhat oxymoronic. What sense does it make to turn a community's development into a service? Doesn't that imply a division between the community and those who are shaping its development? Shouldn't the process of nourishing and developing the vitality of a community be both the responsibility and ambition of its members? Shouldn't theirs be the directing energy behind any new development? Shouldn't they be the agents of desirable change?

Jenny Hartnoll and her team at Health Connections Mendip take such issues seriously. Community development is a component of their work but the aim is to facilitate the process through the autonomous activity of those community members who volunteer as community connectors or serve it as health connectors, along with the inspirational efforts of all the other people who set up the many varied group activities and concerns which give the town and its surrounding area its characteristic vitality.

That vitality derives from the organic manner in which all these different components fit together cohesively and inter-dependently. The mapping of those resources and the ongoing compilation of the service directory have formed a bank of essential information about what the community has to offer. It's a bank on which anyone can freely draw.

The directory was designed for ease of use, but even a well-designed website is of no value to anyone without access to a computer or those whose first language is not English. Face-to-face communication is the key to a healthy community life, and the lively chatter of conversation in the talking cafés creates ample opportunities for spreading useful information by word of mouth. So too do the multiplying number of conversations about things going on in the community that are prompted by community connectors every year. Once the service directory and the talking cafés are in place, the community connectors play a vital role in the overall picture. Their well-trained knowledge of what the directory contains and their ability to access and use that bank of information translates it from inert text into creative action that reaches throughout the whole community.

The combination of these factors opens the doors of possibility by pointing people towards those specific aspects of a wide variety of social resources – interest groups, joint enterprises, offers of reliable support – which may be of interest and concern to them. Rather than pushing people into doing things they don't want to do, it offers encouraging invitations to improve and enrich the quality of their lives by taking advantage of events and activities which afford the kind of company, shared laughter and friendship on which a true sense of belonging is built. And should it become clear that an individual's expressed needs or areas of interest are not covered by what is already on offer in the community, then the development service will look for means to convert that lack into an opportunity to create something new.

KATHY'S STORY

Moving evidence of how a Compassionate Communities programme can be both a healing and a transformative experience is offered by the story of Kathy, whose enviably happy life was devastated by the onset of severe illness and then put back together through her revitalizing involvement in the radically activated social life of Frome.

A married woman in her early fifties with two grown-up sons and a much-loved Labrador dog, Kathy was employed as human resources director for a large company when she developed pain and swelling in her knees and her hands. Initially, Kathy shrugged it off as best she could, thinking she had simply hurt her knee while walking her dog through muddy Somerset fields one morning. But the pain endured and after a visit to the GP and follow-up tests, a diagnosis of rheumatoid arthritis was confirmed. Unfortunately, it was a very aggressive form of the disease and, within the space of three weeks, Kathy's condition worsened to such a degree that she needed a wheelchair simply for getting around:

> I realized that this was not something that was just a short-lived health condition. I heeded the advice that I should stop work but then experienced a very quick spiral downwards. I had to use a mobility scooter and my walking had become very laboured, with the use of crutches. I became very low. It felt like my life had ground to a halt. I went to the GP and admitted how isolated I felt. My husband and boys would be out to work during the day and my house wasn't practical with my mobility issues. I still had my beloved dog, but even he would look at me forlornly, missing the long walks that until only recently we took every day.

Thanks to Health Connections Mendip, part of the blossoming compassion project, Kathy had a life-changing visit from Rose, one of the health connectors. During a tearful hour and a half, Kathy admitted to Rose that what she really needed was to have people around her. She was so used to working with people and being immersed in her busy work and family life that the diagnosis was like a thunderbolt that had struck her down. Kathy knew that life could no longer be the same as before, but she pleaded with Rose: 'I need to know that this is not going to be how I am going to be for the rest of my life.'

Though she could not know it, in that moment Kathy was at the start of a completely unexpected journey which would soon transform her into a woman with a newfound sense of heart and purpose. That journey began with one simple recommendation Rose made after listening to Kathy and giving her the space in which she could ask for help – that she join a group run at the health centre by another health connector, which met fortnightly on Tuesdays.

The group was an 'on track' group for people setting goals for their health and well-being. Kathy immediately took to the can-do nature of the group and also quickly learned about the 'self-management' pain group, a six-week programme, run twice weekly, for the purpose of talking through the process of coming to terms with a chronic illness that was going to last a long time. As well as receiving invaluable guidance on how best to manage the illness both physically and emotionally, Kathy was also made aware of other resources in Frome, such as physiotherapy, hydrotherapy and mindfulness courses. As movement became a little easier, she could get about with a stick rather than having to rely on a wheelchair.

Describing the group, Kathy says:

There were 12 of us in very similar phases of an illness. The doctors had said there was not much more they could do but it was 'about managing your condition, how you rely on your support network and your friends. Don't be afraid to ask for help and learn how to pace yourself.' There were some in the group who had just started their journey and others who had come through the other side. It was a great help, listening to them talk through the experiences that they had had.

Chronic pain is thought to affect at least one-third of adults in the UK and is often part of the same debilitating cycle in which loneliness and isolation are key factors. As Kathy observed, there might be little that doctors can do to cure patients of pain, but gradually, through learning about her disease and about ways to manage her pain, Kathy's daily experience improved measurably. She also attended the 'escaping pain' group, which taught Kathy a sequence of gentle exercises that took into account the physical limitations caused by her rheumatoid arthritis. Attending the group gave her the confidence to know that she could have a life that included exercise. It also encouraged healthy eating and taught her how she could help herself when she suffered a flare-up of her disease.

The next step for Kathy was to start going out into the community.

Jo, the health connector who ran the groups inside the practice, also ran exercise groups out in the community. But the groups are not just limited to exercise. There are art classes, organized walks, the couch to 5k runs (which I can't yet do but am aspiring to do so) and others.

In a process called 'signposting', Kathy now directs people who are currently in a similar position to the one in which she found herself 18 months previously to community resources. She is able to drive again and so helps others to get around. She now works part-time and spends some time in the medical centre as a community connector, making herself available to anyone coming there who might benefit from the kind of help that she herself once badly needed and gratefully received.

Just like the authors of this book, it was a moment of *keraunos* that initially brought Kathy to a low point of despair and need but so began a journey in her life that led to a deep and transformative experience of compassion, so much so that her life's priorities have completely changed and she is now giving back the same powerful medicine of compassion that she received.

I knew my neighbours to wave to. I have never spent time with them. And here I was, suddenly helpless and at home. Without even asking, between them they rallied round. They made sure someone came to see me every day, to see how I was and if there were errands to run. I had never come across this before. My life was focused on my family and my work. My experiences have made me very humble and appreciative. People do actually care. I have become so thankful that there are people willing to help. I have made so many friends. I am now going out into the community, talking to people to say there is hope and they are not alone. People who go through similar experiences become lifelong friends. That is the most important thing I have learnt. I will be there for them and they will be there for me. I've been given my life back.'

THE OBVIOUS

There are, of course, people in similar circumstances to Kathy who do not have the confidence or clarity of mind to know what it is they want, or how to act on it. They may simply be confused by the variety and complexity of what is going on in the community around them. Such people are vital reminders, if any were needed, that the foundational value of the entire Health Connections Mendip enterprise, whether overtly stated or not, is compassion. That is where it begins, that is how it grows, and that is what it creates.

Yet one of the difficulties that presents itself in writing about all this is that so much of it is, frankly, obvious. Do we really need to point out that life would be better for us all if people were simply kind and supportive to one another? Isn't it clearly apparent that a community would be more creatively vibrant, and probably more content, if it took direct responsibility for managing its affairs in a manner governed by a compassionate concern for the happiness and welfare of all its members? And how is it possible that we ever thought a different way of doing things might be better?

Those hard-bitten by their experience of the world might answer that such utopian speculations are merely fanciful and unrealistic. But those who pride themselves on being realists have too often settled for a meaner vision of life and its possibilities. The example of what is being achieved in Frome offers a working model of a feasible alternative. Not that anyone in the town considers it to be utopia – a word which, in any case, means 'nowhere', and in which misplaced political faith has sometimes led to ruin. Like everywhere else, the town has its troubles and its problems, but it also now has a presiding vision and a pragmatic approach to what to do to diminish these problems, a vision that has grown from within rather than as a scheme imposed from above.

That vision is embodied in the work and character of Jenny Hartnoll, of her friend and colleague Dr Helen Kingston, and of the whole team of Health Connections Mendip. In collaboration with the people of the town, they are busy making common sense out of complex issues. Their combination of imaginative forward thinking with an open-minded, practical approach to getting on with the job is proving fruitful.

For them, setting a plan does not mean that everything is fixed and pre-determined. Rather, as a flexible guide to steering community life in what feels like the right direction, while at the same time staying open to new possibilities for development as needs and circumstance arise, the project is making, in troubled times, a strong case for hope.

PART TWO

HARNESSING THE
POWER OF COMPASSION

CHAPTER 6

COMPASSION AND
THE INDIVIDUAL

*I see the world moving in two different directions. The one
promoted by our business and government leaders is toward this
outdated model of growth, pushing harder and harder to expand,
to scale up and speed up that system. In the meanwhile, the earth
is crying out against it, people are crying out against it, and in
virtually every economic forum now there are demonstrations.
The great hope is that from the bottom up people are moving in
exactly the opposite direction, which is toward community.*

Helen Norberg-Hodge

The success of the efforts made by the Compassionate Frome
project suggests that informally available community
resources may hold the key to solving many of the problems
currently afflicting society. And that the building of a compassionate
community begins not with the imposition of an ideology but with
the cultivation of the active power of compassion within individuals.
It begins with cultivating a compassionate life.

There are, of course, many factors that count against such an
optimistic perspective. Social problems have become so severe

in many urban and rural areas of fiercely competitive industrial and commercial societies that it's not unreasonable to question whether compassion can still be considered a widely available resource. Meanwhile, at the individual level, psychological studies of personality, which divide human types into various categories, including both the tough and the tender-minded, might seem to endorse a common assumption that any given individual either has compassion for others or does not. By extension, the further assumption that such a condition is not open to change or development complements the loose division of the human race into grim realists on the one hand and bleeding-heart idealists on the other.

Such commonly held attitudes may be discouraging, but a careful look at what is actually happening in our communities and in our own lives reveals many examples of the compassionate spirit in action. It shows how that spirit already energizes many individuals, while also providing evidence that its influence can be fostered by the power of example.

Such fuller recognition of our own capacity for compassion deepens the understanding that all human beings, irrespective of race, cultural background, personality or any other characteristic, share this same potential. Though it may be active in them to a greater or lesser degree, or at times not active at all, the potential remains, and the awareness that it is possible to activate it calls into question the truth of those pessimistic assertions that human nature is unchangeable. As we have seen, the capacity for compassion has been built into our species through evolution and is present in human biochemistry and physiology. A compassionate response to the world is available to us at every moment.

RECOGNIZING AND ASSESSING OUR OWN COMPASSIONATE RESOURCES

The effort to find and sustain a compassionate response to the difficult, emotionally challenging situations that confront us in our lives is, in effect, a journey into greater consciousness. Such an effort draws us out of our comfort zone by requiring us to comprehend and evaluate issues and experiences from points of view other than our own. It also demands a clear-sighted acknowledgement of our own limitations and the employment of appropriate strategies to help us deal with them creatively. Compassion isn't only the wish to alleviate suffering; it is pragmatic and practical, it demands action. This is often where individuals might feel powerless or may struggle with the de-energizing effects of compassion fatigue: there is just too much suffering to know where to begin. But the power of compassion doesn't change the world in one great step. It begins with the people who are sitting next to us.

A considered awareness of our own strengths and weaknesses helps to keep our expectations realistic and thus decreases the chances of finding ourselves disheartened by failure to achieve overly ambitious goals. To that point, it's as well to remember that such avatars of compassion as Gautama Buddha, Mahatma Gandhi and Martin Luther King were very rare figures indeed. The same is true of such profoundly empathetic women as Beatrice Webb, who gave up her comfortable bourgeois life to work in a textile factory in order to experience and draw attention to the hardships faced by the destitute working class, and the product designer Patricia Moore, who, at age 26, visited North American cities for three years disguised as an 85-year-old woman suffering from various disabilities in order to identify the many physical problems faced by the elderly in a largely indifferent world.

Compassionate action is beneficial for everyone, everywhere, but for it to become truly effective each of us has to arrive at that conclusion for ourselves. Once that understanding is achieved then compassion becomes a principal source of motivation in our daily lives. This amounts to more than a matter of not doing harm. It is an active not a passive stance and wherever there is interaction between humans and whenever decisions are made which affect lives, active compassion becomes a positively transformative force. Think of Kathy, whose outlook on life was transformed, first by the compassion that was shown to her just at the moment she needed it, and now by the way in which she offers her own experience as a compassionate helping hand to others.

Furthermore, we have to start recognizing that there is something sadly wrong with people who seem incapable of compassion. There is an aberration in their character which can have deeply harmful consequences for themselves and others. A terrifying – though extreme – example of this is provided by a sign that hung above the desk of Hans Stark, the head of the admissions detail at Auschwitz. It said simply *Mitleid ist Schwache*, advising his subordinates that 'compassion is weakness'. This reminds us that a lack of compassion is not simply a neutral act: it is an active choice which has the potential to cause harm.

Compassion is an uncomfortable feeling because it refuses to turn away from the suffering of others and lets it weigh on the heart. By contrast, hardening our hearts to the plight of others allows us to abandon them and abnegate responsibility. A move towards the evolution of a more compassionate society will depend on individuals working for such change in their own behaviour.

There is good scientific evidence that physiological change takes place in individuals who develop the practice of compassion. Studies have shown that people who volunteer have lower rates of mortality, and volunteers who suffer from chronic health conditions or disabilities themselves often experience an improvement in their symptoms after giving their time to help others. Psychopathic individuals and children who have suffered abuse often have smaller amygdalae than others – the part of the brain that plays a key role in the processing of emotions – but as they learn to develop compassion that almond-shaped grouping of neurons increases in size.

PRACTISING COMPASSION

To live life as a compassion project requires that one does not turn away from another's suffering but relates to it creatively. It asks that attention be given both to the grief of the world and to that of those immediately around us, by taking time to listen, for example, or simply by remaining present. And it also demands an active readiness to help those in need in whatever ways our individual capacities permit.

It is perhaps easier to respond to suffering with feelings of shame or guilt, but by nurturing compassion we may be inspired to act upon, rather than avoid, what is in front of us. A conscious commitment to small acts of compassionate behaviour can have a significant effect on both the quality of other people's lives and on our feelings about ourselves. As well as the immediate one-to-one exchange of benevolent energy, they have a knock-on effect on the enhancement of community life. People begin to take a more active interest in each other's welfare through caring enquiries and positive response; shopping becomes a social event rather than a merely commercial transaction; kinder interactions take place at work and there is a greater willingness to engage with strangers in a friendly, less defensive manner.

Julian recalls an incident that took place in a supermarket where a saxophonist was playing along to Christmas songs.

As we arrived at the checkout, the tune playing was 'Lonely This Christmas'. The woman serving us at the counter had a tear in her eye. We asked her why and she said her son had died recently. As death is unusual in a younger person, I asked what her son had died from and she replied that he had taken his own life. This was such a touching and immensely sad moment. It was easy to understand why she felt tearful at this first Christmas without her son. It was a brief but meaningful interaction, touched with simple compassion, and I'm glad we were able to be kind to her.

MINDFULNESS AND COMPASSION

At the heart of finding the patience and presence to be compassionate with others lies the ability to feel true compassion for oneself. Use of the rational mind may help us to recognize, in theory at least, that all humans have the inbuilt potential for compassion, but engagement of more than the rational mind is needed if that is to be realized. In Buddhist traditions, the purpose of the practice of meditation is to bring forth the recognition of our innate compassion and wisdom. This is the direct experience of our compassionate nature, present in all of us as a potential and realized to a greater or lesser extent.

The human mind is constantly distracted and agitated by the thoughts and emotions that pass through it with sometimes overwhelming speed and intensity. We are all familiar with the way that even relatively tranquil states of mind can very quickly be disturbed by complex associations and memories, along with doubts of self-worth, all of them often deeply rooted in personal history and re-activated by immediate experience.

The meditation known as calm abiding is an effective method of allaying such turbulent emotions by holding one's focus on a particular object and bringing the attention back to that focus when it strays. The selected object may be internal – the breathing process or a visualized image – or external in the form, for example, of a conveniently placed piece of wood or stone. The effectiveness of the method relies on the use of the two related faculties of mindfulness and awareness.

Mindfulness allows us to remember to remain focused on the object of meditation. Thus, when focusing on the movement of the breath in and out of the body, one can remain mindful by counting the number of breaths up to seven, for example, or on to twenty-one or more depending on how skilful we are at focusing and remembering to keep count.

Awareness is the faculty which determines whether our minds are suffering from the two major obstacles to sustained meditation. The first obstacle is that of dullness – the tendency of the mind to become heavy and drowsy, even to fall asleep when, for example, counting the numbers of breath cycles. The remedy for this is to sit upright and tighten one's awareness by refocusing. The second obstacle to meditation is that of mental agitation when our thoughts accelerate and disturb our tranquillity. With mindfulness in place, we use our awareness to determine whether the mind has lost focus and begun to rush. The remedy is to relax one's posture a little and thus also relax the mind.

Inevitably, our minds wander as our mindfulness and awareness wane, and it is part of the meditation process to re-establish their strength. When the mind strays, one simply notices and brings it back into focus without passing judgement and carries on with the meditation. One learns in this way to let go of the torrents of thought that disturb our peace and thus gradually train the mind to replace the monkey-like habits of mental distraction with that of sustained focus. The essential quality of this focus is a balanced awareness which is neither too heavy nor too active. In this way, it becomes increasingly possible to keep awareness sharp and bright while remaining mentally relaxed.

A routine practice of meditation which starts with short bursts that last for just a few minutes, either daily or a number of times each day, reduces the chance of becoming overwhelmed by the demands of the process or disappointed if progress feels slow. The aim is to let the mind relax in a focused way that allows some breathing space from the rough and tumble of daily existence. A relaxed mind gives a sense of inner peace which will permit us to cope more calmly with the challenges of living a compassionate life.

MEDITATIONS TO DEVELOP COMPASSION

In addition to calming the mind, other modes of meditation can help to develop and refine the quality of compassion.

Whether religious or not, many of us tend to pray for help in stressful times, but a more concentrated commitment to prayer is itself a form of meditative practice which heightens receptivity to sources of inspiration and support, both inward and outer, which can help to make our responses kinder and more compassionate.

As has already been pointed out, a vital aspect of compassion is the activity of the sympathetic imagination and its capacity for therapeutic visualization can be used to enhance the quality of compassion. One might, for example, create an inward image of compassion in the embodied form of an inspirational figure radiating waves of compassion across the universe. Such an embodied image might be visualized, according to one's cultural predisposition, as Christ or Buddha, as Allah the All Merciful or as Kuan Yin, the Goddess of Compassion. Or one might choose to imagine compassion as a radiating ball of light encompassing the darkness without limitation. Whatever the form of the image, its light should be imagined entering the body, suffusing it and washing away those negative beliefs, ideas and emotions which impede the flow of compassion. And not just compassion for others but also for ourselves, for self-compassion – which can be a profoundly emotional experience – is necessary if we are to activate our full compassionate potential.

We all make mistakes at times and behave in ways of which we may be far from proud, especially if we have caused harm to others. At such moments the thought of forgiving oneself for what is in fact very human behaviour may be far from one's mind, but the use of a method of meditation that helps us to acknowledge and then forgive our faults can bring forth genuine feelings of regret. Though those feelings may be distressing, a truly mindful process of contrition can strengthen us to put self-defeating negative emotions behind us and clear the way for a whole-hearted return to our better nature. Such meditative acts of self-forgiveness require both acknowledgement of what we have done and greater appreciation for what we have. Additionally, meditation offers an incentive to explore those perspectives further and to expand their reach.

Such practices may seem far removed from one's usual approach to everyday life, but mindfulness simply encourages us to pay more careful attention to what actually goes on in daily life. The transformative effects of such attention can be seen both in Jenny Hartnoll's remarkable ability to identify every social resource available in Frome, and in Kathy's journey from despair at loss of her independence to a newfound sense of purpose and increased appreciation of the people in her community. Meditation also encourages us to listen attentively to others rather than sit thinking about what we will say next, and it can help us to alleviate our own anxieties, freeing up our compassion for ourselves, for others, and for the world around us.

In a society where fear is cultivated in order to increase mistrust and where divisions are rife, learning how to calm the mind in this way and open the heart to its essential humankindness can help to transform the prevailing feel of the world. For a growing certainty that the capacity for compassion can be strengthened will generate the necessary confidence to convert what might otherwise be little more than noble aspirations into beneficent and socially effective action.

FACING CHALLENGES TO OUR COMPASSION

But the fact is that we all have our own limitations. So it's not surprising if we feel our compassion flag when we endure periods of emotional conflict, exhaustion and distress. Or that things tend to go awry when we ask too much of ourselves, or a situation. In these situations, meditation alone may not be enough to get us back on track and we may need to turn to other sources of help.

For some people, making a vow – whether religious or not – can help to reinvigorate commitment and remind us of our original purpose in the toughest of times. This is, of course, the reason why the rituals of marriage institute solemn vows as the foundation for a lifelong commitment. When pressure builds to breaking point and a carer's sense of frustration and impatience burn more strongly than their love and compassion, the vow not only acts as a reminder of that commitment, it can provide a source of strength to honour it. However, a vow has to be based on realistic expectations determined by self-knowledge, and the ability to keep it over a long period of time will depend on sustained efforts of self-discipline.

There is also the danger that failing to stick to a resolution such as this will deepen feelings of guilt, adding to the overall stress of the situation, so it makes sense to develop a strategy of what to do when the vow weakens.

Generally speaking, it's important to take periodic breaks from the pressure of trying to be a good carer or simply meeting the demands of living a compassionate life. Too commonly, people tend to put their own pleasures and interests aside as they focus on the demands of caring for a loved one. But, as we have seen, engaging in enjoyably distracting activities can provide restorative periods of rest from incessant anxious thoughts, whether that's spending time with friends, sports, games, a long solitary walk or run. Whatever the preference, simply doing something pleasurably different from the demands of the usual routine will enhance one's resilience and strengthen the fortitude to cope well with one's responsibilities.

In short, an essential aspect of making compassion a fundamental principle of one's life is the ability to be compassionate with oneself, and to do that in a way which, as far as possible, keeps the heart open and warm in relation to others.

Sooner or later, the chances are that most, if not all, of us will need help in coping with tormenting negative emotions that oppress our minds and hearts, making it difficult for us to feel much in the way of active compassion for others. The first port of call in such unhappy circumstances might be a member of the family or a trusted friend, but sometimes it can be far from easy to speak truthfully or completely to people who may themselves be party to the problem. In this situation it may be necessary to speak to a professional psychotherapeutic service. For many people, the techniques taught by cognitive behavioural therapy (CBT) can be employed as an effective aid in examining habituated responses and the accompanying negative emotions. Once it is realized that a given mode of thought need not lead to an inevitable set of consequences, a larger degree of change becomes possible.

The power of self-sabotaging thoughts can be diminished by such a shift of perspective, and there are many other, deeper searching forms of psychotherapeutic practice which, through careful examination of lived experience, often over many sessions, can assist clients to evaluate and correct faulty perceptions, to convert negative emotions into creative energy and to draw on the transformative resources of the unconscious mind. In all these ways the capacity for truly grounded compassion can be cultivated.

Giving help and support to someone in need is effective and rewarding to the degree that it is informed by genuine feelings of compassion. So in that respect it's important to remember the need to have compassion for ourselves as well as others. Caring for someone is stressful. Emotions can easily get frayed, especially if we are tired and struggling to cope with loss and the changes happening around us. Even in good, longstanding relationships such stress can exacerbate feelings of impatience and irritation, and failure to respect the limits of one's own resources can lead to illness, which will render us useless to anyone. In such circumstances, a mutually compassionate acknowledgement that we might be overly sensitive to one another's actions and reactions can mitigate the stress.

It's important also to understand that there is a significant difference between freely offered care and care given in expectation of receiving something in return. If we give as some kind of transactional exchange, whether monetary or through some other contract such as those of the time-bank schemes in which communities exchange goods or services, the giving is commodified. Though we may feel good about what we give, a specific valuation has been placed on the quality of the gift and this brings its own expectations. In turn, these can lead to disappointment or resentment.

The story of sad events in Madagascar during the 1980s graphically illustrates this point. A voluntary literacy programme freely conceived and staffed by literate members of a local community became so popular and successful with those suffering from the disadvantages of illiteracy that international aid agencies decided to fund the work by paying a wage to the teachers. At that point the programme collapsed.

Why did that happen? Because once monetary value had been placed on their efforts, the volunteers elected to stop teaching until they were paid what they considered to be suitable amounts of money for their work. By contrast, their original unconditional offer of help raised no questions of valuation or return. The shots of oxytocin released by such altruistic motivation made the volunteers feel good, and the knowledge that they were doing a fine thing was its own reward. Ironically, the introduction of payment to support those efforts literally put paid to them.

THE POWER OF INSPIRATION

The creative activity of the imagination is a potent source of compassionate energy. The imagination has two aspects: the inventive or poetic aspect, which conceives and finds expressive form, and the sympathetic or ethical aspect, which allows us to perceive, recognize and respect reality from points of view other than our own. Without the ethical aspect, the activity of the imagination can generate ideas, images and stories (that of Hitler's 'master race' for example) which are pernicious and destructive in their effects. And if the ethical aspect loses touch with the poetic, it can be overly cerebral, didactic and propagandist. But when the two aspects work fruitfully together, what the imagination produces can touch head, heart and soul in ways that enhance and enlarge our sense of what is true and real. And because of that, its effects – the way it moves us – can be transformative.

This was well understood in the ancient world. Aristotle articulated the idea that the impact on the audience of a great tragic play was cathartic – which is to say that it required them to suffer vicariously the anguish of the characters in the drama, and thus drew their consciousness beyond its normal range of egoic preoccupation.

The same understanding has underpinned the initiatory rites of traditional peoples across the globe. When asked by an anthropologist about the role of story in the life of his tribe, the Apache Indian Benton Lewis uttered three apparently simple sentences: 'Stories go to work on you like arrows. Stories make you live right. Stories make you replace yourself.' If one were to translate into ideas what were, for him, experiences, they might read something like this:

Firstly, that when one hears or reads a truly good story it pierces you to the heart; it can make you feel pain in both body and mind; it can shake and stun you into immediate recognition that something important and penetrating has happened to you.

Secondly, that a story rightly told has ethical value because it can make you question the implications, and even the foundations, of the way in which you are living your life and perhaps also strive to correct them.

And finally, that the experience can prove so deeply transformative that, when the story has ended, the reader or listener is no longer quite the same person that they were when the story began, and that change may be radical.

All three of Benton Lewis's statements endorse, from a timeless traditional perspective, the thinking behind E M Forster's belief that, 'If human nature does alter it will be because individuals manage to look at themselves in a new way.' Not only can they be read as affirmations of the power of the compassionate imagination in human life, they are also salutary reminders that reading fiction is more than a passive mode of entertainment – it is itself an activity of the imagination which has participatory effect and can have moral consequence. Out of the black words on the white page, readers are provoked to create for themselves the characters and events of the story and to inhabit their world. In so doing, they have scope to widen their own perspectives and to nourish their capacity for compassion in what can be inspiring ways.

The transformative power of love and compassion, and the tragic effects of their absence, have always been among the major themes of great art in poetry, novels, opera, drama and films. Such enduring works carry ethical as well as aesthetic value. Thus, to accompany King Lear across the storm-blown heath and suffer along with him as his proud and purblind heart finally learns to feel for those around him is to undergo a painful rite of initiation into greater consciousness. To contemplate Wolfram von Eschenbach's marvellous version of the story of the Grail is to journey with its hero Parzival as he crosses a waste land ravaged by the masculine quest for power and glory to discover at last that it can only be made green again by the active power of human compassion. And to read George Eliot's magnificent novel *Middlemarch* is to learn how to be compassionate with the hopes and griefs, trials and tribulations of ordinary men and women living out their lives in a quiet provincial town, and be assured that, in the final words of the novel, 'The growing good of the world is partly dependent on unhistoric acts; and that things are not so ill with you and me as they might have been is half owing to the number who lived faithfully a hidden life, and rest in unvisited tombs.'

For the imagination to engage deeply with such works is to undergo what Gaston Bachelard called 'a homeopathy of anguish', effectively educating us in life's ambiguities, lending larger dimensions of recognition, value and meaning to our own lived experiences and – importantly – giving us a flavour of anguish so that we may be prepared for it when it arrives.

Of course, such demanding works of literature are not to everybody's taste, but the elemental wisdom that makes them endure has a way of percolating through to popular culture via other media. Consider the way, for example, that the stage version, and later the film, of *West Side Story* drew on the narrative and imagery of Shakespeare's *Romeo and Juliet* to make an impact on the contemporary heart by drawing on the combined power of music, song and dance. Similarly, Francis Ford Coppola's film *Apocalypse Now* offered an updated version of Joseph Conrad's excoriating novella *Heart of Darkness* to confront its audience with the depraved insanity of the Vietnam War. It's a film that arouses pity and fear in truly cathartic manner and therefore can work transformative effect. More recently, even as audiences to the film *Capernaum* bear witness to the plight of children on the war-ravaged streets of Lebanon, their hearts are moved and uplifted by the way those children are still able to express love and kindness to each other despite the daily brutality and hardship they endure.

Such experiences of the power of story can be inspirational and it's highly significant that, in times of loss and distress, many people – including those with no particular interest in literature or any other form of art – will turn to poetry for consolation. It's as if, almost instinctively, they are drawn to it as a source of healing and recuperation. Perhaps it's for this reason that Neil Astley's fine anthologies of verse, *Being Alive* and *Staying Alive,* have enjoyed such widespread attention. By ordering a wide variety of poems by many different poets in a manner that addresses the major areas of experience such collections offer to a largely secular age the kind of insight, guidance and comfort that was once commonly sought in religious texts, as well as displaying the wit and verve of human intelligence. Perhaps most importantly, they also strengthen the faith that even bewildering events in our lives can be made intelligible to heart and mind through the ordering powers of language and imagination.

In a time of accelerating environmental crisis, it should also be urgently said that, perhaps more intimately than any other art form, though with the wordless exception of music, poetry can alert us to the voice of what William Wordsworth called 'the Wisdom and Spirit of the Universe'. Its images and rhythms can remind us that our little human lives are part of a far vaster scheme of life that is animate and active everywhere around us, and which we demean and degrade at our peril.

Many poets attribute the authority of their verse to a source beyond themselves – 'Not I, but the wind that blows through me,' is how D H Lawrence expressed it. To do this is to acknowledge the wider inspirational power of the natural order. Wordsworth was another poet whose work is rooted in the power and stimulation offered by landscape and the natural word. In his *Lines Composed a Few Miles above Tintern Abbey,* he celebrates the power of nature as an inspiration and a guide, and reflects on the inter-connectedness of all things:

> *A presence that disturbs me with the joy*
> *Of elevated thoughts; a sense sublime*
> *Of something far more deeply interfused,*

Whose dwelling is the light of setting suns,
And the round ocean and the living air,
And the blue sky, and in the mind of man:
A motion and a spirit that impels,
All thinking things, all objects of all thought,
And rolls through all things.

It is in his vision of the natural world that Wordsworth hears, 'the still sad music of humanity,' for that is where our species deeply belongs. We are inseparably a part of it all and it is where our physical and spiritual being is most clearly nourished and refreshed. When given our proper attention, it is also, for all of us, an unfailing source of creative inspiration.

Through daily mindful acts of care, however small, we will help to correct disabling negative assumptions about our own nature and build confidence that we are capable of changing things for the better, both inside ourselves and for the sake of the world around us. That is what it can mean to regard one's individual life as a compassion project.

CHAPTER 7

WEAVING COMPASSIONATE
NETWORKS

We need to take action to develop compassion, to create inner peace within ourselves and to share that inner peace with our family and friends. Peace and warm-heartedness can then spread through the community just as ripples radiate out across the water when you drop a pebble into a pond.

Dalai Lama XIV

Though we identify ourselves as individuals, we actually live in the plural. We are interdependent beings cared for by the people around us who form those networks of relationship that provide us with support, companionship and the basic necessities of life. The success of the Compassionate Frome project stemmed in large measure from an initial awareness of the vital importance of these networks in our lives, and then from the way it publicized and promoted the existing web of supportive relationships already active in the town and set about creating more of them to meet newly recognized needs.

Because their true value is not always fully appreciated, this chapter will take a closer look at the intricately networked patterns of relationships, familial and tribal, which have been built into the way we live through millions of years of evolution. Though they may vary in form and customs, the bonding power that holds them together is – at their heart – our innate human capacity for kindness and compassion.

Our health and welfare depend on these networks for the essential support we need. For that reason, as we have already seen, a person suffering from a poverty of social contact is more likely to die prematurely. For the same reason, solitary confinement can be used as a form of torture because most people fall apart psychologically when deprived for long periods of the company of others.

Though we tend to take the importance of warm social interaction for granted, a moment's thought can remind us that we value the members of our various supportive networks not just because they prove helpful in times of trouble, but because we have deep, life-affirming feelings towards people who endorse and enrich our sense of personal identity.

In short, because they make us feel good.

SOCIAL RELATIONSHIPS AND IDENTITY

In a world constantly busy with other preoccupations, it can be easy to underestimate the importance of the casual, day-to-day interactions we have with those around us. Though we may value the people close to us for their warmth, for their love and friendship they share with us, for their willingness to talk freely and hear what we have to say, for the small acts of kindness they show, or simply because they are such good fun that it's a joy to be in their company – we may still fail to appreciate how, piece by piece, our interactions with them contribute to our health and welfare, and our sense of personal identity. Whether members of our family, friends or just congenial people we come across in our daily life, their presence is part of the positive feedback that makes us feel at home in the world. They affirm our sense of belonging and, when we think about them, we value them not for what they do but for who they are.

By contrast, when we think about ourselves it can be a different matter, particularly when we feel confused, undervalued or threatened. We tend to base our judgement less on the particular qualities of the person we feel we are than on the character, successful or otherwise, of what it is that we do. Thus, our career status can play a large part in defining our identity.

Driven by internalized parental expectations or the demands of societal pressure, some people devote their lives less to fostering mature relationships than to acquiring conspicuous displays of wealth or other visible signals of worldly fame, status and power. Often enough those ambitions can prove destructive both to those who hold them or to the people around them, while any positive feedback gained through sycophantic friendships based on material values differs greatly in its quality and effects from the rewards of truly human love and as a substantial foundation for identity it is much less secure.

By the same token, if we are unemployed or are defined by menial work which is tiring, unsatisfying or poorly paid, our self-esteem may diminish until depression sets in. This can put a strain on friendships, leading to a sense of social isolation and perhaps to the transient comforts of addiction, which can then accelerate a decline in physical and mental health. Whether or not we enjoy our work, if the fatigue of illness – physical or mental – makes it difficult to perform the professional or domestic tasks that have come to define our identity, then our sense of personal worth is further degraded. To judge ourselves by our frailties and failures in this respect may leave us feeling that we have become little more than a burden to those around us. Such feelings of worthlessness can lead to desperation.

When we take the time to consider our interdependence with the world around us, it becomes clear that aggressive individualism is rarely the source of happiness and contentment. Once we fully appreciate the degree to which the people around us meet our deep needs for companionship, collaboration and connection, we can see that compassion is an essential ingredient of a good life. Consciously or otherwise, compassion is at the heart of the human experience and the loss of contact with it can be severe enough to cause early death or have other devastating impacts. The book *Romania's Abandoned Children: Deprivation, Brain Development, and the Struggle for Recovery* by Charles Nelson of Harvard Medical School records a decade-long study of how, in contrast to the children who were allocated to foster care, those remaining in state institutions suffered severe impairment of brain development and intelligence levels as well as a variety of emotional and social disorders. Meanwhile, in our own society, the evidence is that the recent alarming rise in knife crime among the young can be traced back to chaotic parenting in environments of severe economic and social deprivation.

The close support of family, friends and community is the foundation of a healthy worthwhile life and it is through the compassionate development of those relationships that we can both strengthen an authentic sense of personal identity and improve the quality of life in the wider world.

NETWORKS OF RELATIONSHIPS

The proliferation of online communication between people who may meet rarely or even not at all has led to a somewhat diminished meaning of the term 'social network', while in competitive professional circles 'networking' tends to be associated with the purpose-driven quest for influence and career advancement. Yet it is through living webs of social relationship that we have always shaped our individual sense of the world we inhabit.

Though the number of people in those networks may vary according to our personalities and circumstances, their patterns fall into two general categories: an inner network of those to whom we feel most closely attached and an outer network consisting both of people we know well and those with whom we have lighter, less frequent contact. Beyond those networks lies the larger community to which we belong – the village, town or city in which we live. Thus, a diagram of our expanding pattern of networks looks like this:

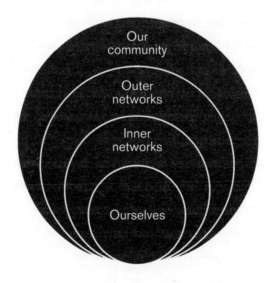

Although these distinct patterns exist, they are not fixed in their form and there are no strict boundaries or rules governing membership. We constantly make choices about how close or distant we feel towards people and those choices may change, allowing for a flow of movement between the networks.

Inner networks

Those people who are closest to us might be family members, friends, neighbours or work colleagues, and we might also include our dogs, cats and other pets. There are no objective rules about how wide our inner network may be or who qualifies for inclusion. Much depends on our personality and lifestyle, so the nature of inner networks varies from individual to individual. The network may have two members or twenty, and a large network is not necessarily more beneficial than a smaller, more intimate one. Neither is geographical proximity a limit. Some of us have family members on the other side of the world with whom we are able to talk regularly via such online media as Facetime and Skype. Those means of communication may not be as intimate as immediate face-to-face contact, but they still enable us to judge the impact on others of what we say to them and then to respond to it with a degree of sensitivity.

Because it is so close to us, the membership of our inner network is easily taken for granted, except of course in times of emergency. But its importance to our welfare and general morale cannot be overstated. In sickness or in health, through good times and hard, a carefully maintained inner network is both the matrix and guarantor of our well-being.

It may seem rather obvious to state the importance of our inner network, and yet such are the societal pressures to feel that we are not a 'burden' to our loved ones that too many people today feel that suffering alone or even ending their life would be preferable for all. Dr Julian Abel worked for over two decades as a palliative care physician, looking after people who were dying and at the same time showing care for their families. He says:

Throughout my clinical practice, people have asked me to help them to end their life, but I cannot remember a single person asking me to help them to die because of unbearable physical suffering. Rather, these requests have been because people have lost their sense of personal value and identity. They feel they are a burden to those around them and they are no longer able to maintain who they feel they are through what they do.

In her wise book on the challenges and positive discoveries of ageing, *Warmth of the Heart Prevents Your Body from Rusting*, the psychologist Marie de Hennezel reflects on the story of a biologist who decided to end her days by suicide. Asked by a journalist if she was depriving her children of the end of her life, the woman replied, 'Deprive? What does that mean? What would it give to them? They have their own lives, their cares, their families.' De Hennezel comments, 'These words reveal more than just a woman's simple desire to control her death. They suggest that her end concerns no one but her...How sad that elderly people do not realize that by experiencing their death in the presence of their loved ones, they communicate something precious. They show them that human beings are capable of accomplishing this act of life.'

Julian Abel tells a similar story:

I remember a man suffering from motor neurone disease who, even though his daughters and those around him loved him for who he was, committed suicide at the point when he needed help to go to the toilet. In those times, when people feel that their life is worthless, I discuss questions of meaning and value with them and ask them to consider how we judge ourselves differently from the way we value others. I try to remind them that the people around us love us for who we are, not for what we do, just as we love and value others in the same way. That they want to spend time with us because they enjoy our company, and those moments of love and friendship can become even more precious when time is limited. In trying to address their sense of loss of value and meaning in life, we would talk about who we love and why we love them. Sometimes I would give people an exercise, asking them to consider what it is that we admire in others and then get them to think about what others admire in them. The aim was to help them reach an understanding of the truth uttered by Cecily Saunders, the founder of the modern palliative medicine movement, when she said, 'You are valuable because you are you'.

Outer networks

Our outer network consists of those acquaintances whom we would not regard as members of the inner network. It may include more distant family relatives along with other friends, work colleagues, neighbours and people with whom we commonly interact in a casual, informal way. We might extend this group to include the postman we chat to, the pharmacist from whom we pick up medicines, the people in shops we often visit and others we occasionally meet.

Julian Abel recalls how he gained a fuller understanding of the importance of these light contacts after listening to a colleague talk about the death of her mother. Her parents moved in with her when her mother became frail. Although this meant hard work, particularly as she had a very busy job and teenage children to care for, she valued her parents and was glad to be able to look after them. About 18 months later, her mother died and, quite soon after the funeral, she went shopping with her father. As they passed from shop to shop, the shopkeepers and people at the supermarket checkout said to her father how sorry they were to hear about his loss, as did the park keeper when they walked in the local park. 'It was clear to my colleague,' says Julian, 'that her parents had developed light but warm and meaningful relationships with the people around them in the city where they had only recently come to live.'

Among the most significant aspects of such relationships can be the sense of pleasant companionship that is generated along the way while we are busy doing something else. In that respect, communal activities such as those of a choir have particular importance. To join a choir is to participate in the joyful and healthy activity of singing, but it also creates valuable opportunities to form new friendships among those who gather to sing. Because choirs often sing together for many years, the members get to know one another well and their meetings can provide affirmative support in a variety of ways at times of need. Even simply expressed words of care from a supportive group can make a tremendous difference at such difficult moments.

Julian Abel reports how he attended a social gathering with his partner who had joined a new choir:

One of the members had lost his wife a year previously. He provided a lift to choir practice to his neighbour and, in this way, she could keep a caring eye on him. I was also struck by the quality of the friendships of the people in the choir. Quite a few of them were single as a result of divorce or bereavement and the friendships created through regular social contact were clearly important to them.

This is just one example of the many ways in which the value of our outer network can expand into something larger and more substantial than we may originally have imagined. If people take full account of the wider pattern of their lives, they often begin to see how what they had considered to be a relatively small group actually consists of as many as fifty, a hundred, or even more people. When we combine the membership of the outer network with the number of those providing us with comfort and kindness in the inner network, we can begin to appreciate that, in terms of the human resources available to us, we may be very wealthy indeed. And beyond that circle are the members of the caring professions and other services on whose help we are free to call in time of need.

The number expands still further when one considers that each person in our networks has their own inner and outer networks of friendship and support to call upon to assist both themselves and others. Furthermore, it is claimed that only six degrees of separation stand between each of us and every other human being on the planet. This means that, starting from someone already known, two people in any part of the world can be linked together by just six separate connecting steps. So, whether or not we appreciate it, we are connected through our compassion. It is as important to us as food and drink, and our very survival ultimately depends upon it.

In his work as a palliative care physician, Julian frequently heard of people living alone with no one to support them, and professional help was therefore presumed essential for their survival. 'If such a person was truly alone, as on a remote island,' he says, 'they couldn't survive, but it's possible that professionals who say that of a person are failing to recognize the available potential of the inner and outer networks in that person's life.'

Of course, not everyone in our networks is going to be a willing helper when support is needed, but the proportion of people who are prepared to help is usually large. Once we know what kind of help is needed, we can overcome any inward resistance to mobilize appropriate networks of support. In that way, one is also contributing to the building of a more compassionate community. But there are many different circumstances in which such needs arise, so we need to consider the varying ways in which networks can work well for us.

SUPPORT FOR THE LONELY

Even if there are people around us and we are physically well, loneliness can have seriously debilitating effects at any time in our lives. Julian recalls a story he heard during a course of network-enhancement training. At one point, participants on the course were asked to think about their own personal network and consider its importance to them.

> *A member of the group talked about how she had moved with her husband from another country to England for work experience. When they first moved, she worked about 90 minutes away from the town where they lived and her husband had to be away from home during the working week. Although she had colleagues at work, she felt very isolated because she had little other contact with people around her. After six weeks this arrangement became unbearable to her. The couple found different jobs and moved to a small village in Scotland, where the social environment proved much less isolating than that of a busy town.*

Access to webs of supportive relationships clearly plays a vital role in our general well-being. Because we benefit from the fluent process of give and take by which they function, it's important to consider the ways in which we can contribute to the vitality of our own networks in the course of our daily lives. Once again, the key factor is compassion. Whether overtly recognized or not, it's the glue that holds networks together and keeps them functioning. By acting out of genuine concern for others, we are able to form firm friendships which strengthen a communal sense of shared interests and shared values.

The sense of identity we gain from such approaches, alongside the affirmative responses of people around us, is a fundamental human need so strong that some of us choose membership of an ultimately self-destructive network of crime, violence and drugs rather than have to endure the isolation of living without a circle of comrades and friends. Disenfranchised teenagers provide a worrying example of such behaviour.

Growing up is a process of gradual separation from our parents as we become increasingly inquisitive about the world and trying to figure out what is important to us commonly leads to a questioning of our parents' values. When that provokes defiant behaviour and discord at home, teenagers may look for a sense of personal identity through joining groups of friends of whom their parents disapprove. This has always been the case, but in today's fragmented urban society, with its increasingly uncertain scale of values, unprecedented numbers of young people are experiencing mental health problems from loneliness and related feelings of exclusion which lead them to join gangs in their search for companionship, identity and self-validation. There are so many examples of ways in which inner city young people can become engaged, such as boxing gyms, martial arts clubs and projects like

RunDemCrew – which in the guise of a simple running club gives young people access to mentoring and advice as well as a safe and unique way to explore London. A compassionate community will be aware of and make best use of all of these things, creating more as the need arises.

More positively, there are, of course, many group activities through which we find an affirmative commonality with others – supporters' clubs for sporting teams, walking groups, the University of the Third Age, craft workshops and book clubs, to name just a few examples. Throughout our lives we seek the convivial warmth, good humour and pleasure that such shared activities can provide. At the end of our days, we may even use them as the standard of whether or not we have lived a worthwhile life.

Whatever their particular focus of interest, what matters most about such social webs of support are the friendships formed along the way. Those friendships are based in feelings of fellowship of which the deep ground is compassion – that sensitive willingness to engage emotionally with the life and welfare of others without which no deeply satisfying and truly meaningful relationships are possible.

COMPASSIONATE SUPPORTIVE NETWORKS AND ILL HEALTH

If social networks are important to us when we are functioning happily and well, they become even more so during times when life confronts us with its harsher challenges. In talking to professionals about issues of ill health, one frequently encounters a revealing assumption that some form of physical support is the kind of help that a patient will need – as if the only thing that matters is the patient's physical welfare. But professionals tend to focus on the deficits they see and conclude that the only people with the know-how to remedy them are the professionals themselves. In this way, the diagnosis of disease and its correct treatment can become all important for a doctor. The belief that the patient couldn't survive without the doctor's intervention relates to the notion of the professional as a hero, as the one who knows the solution. Yet research has shown us that, where longevity is concerned, the health benefits of good relationships can be more effective than any medicine a doctor might prescribe.

When healthcare professionals restrict their ideas about appropriate help to the skilled attention of doctors and the hands-on care of nursing staff, they may be missing the practical importance of an invaluable resource which is among the most powerful medicines at our fingertips. Instead of invoking the patient's caring network as a primary resource in the situation, they reach for pharmaceuticals, which may cause more harm than good in the longer term, and then look to the staff of hospitals and nursing homes to solve the problem of care. There are obviously circumstances in which such institutions will indeed offer the appropriate solution, but the remarkable outcomes of the Compassionate Frome project demonstrate that the best results emerge when all these forms of support work in harmony together. By contrast, it is a regrettably lost opportunity when professionals fail to see, and therefore make no use of, an almost magical social elixir which can prolong life and is available everywhere.

And those beneficent resources are not only important to the patient – they are also needed by members of the supportive network. The resilience of that network is the critical factor in changing the outcomes for people afflicted by ill health. This means that carefully focussed attention on the supportive network should be a routine part of the assessment of the patient's condition.

The overwhelming experience of those suffering from severe illness is that of fatigue. Whether the illness is physical or mental, the depletion of energy that is fatigue leads to restricted mobility and reduced social contact and it is that condition that frequently precipitates a visit to the doctor.

One of the key principles of palliative care in particular, as of healthcare as a whole, is the provision of treatment for the distressing symptoms suffered by patients. Professionals take pride in their ability to alleviate their painful effects but the fatigue that accompanies nearly all ill health is one of the most difficult and debilitating symptoms and, once the illness is advanced, no adequate treatment may be available for it. Many of the medications used to treat other symptoms, such as pain or nausea and vomiting, have the side-effect of aggravating energy loss and fatigue. The consequential loss of social function can then create serious existential problems.

Once people feel unable to relate to those around them, their sense of meaning and value can deteriorate to such a degree that they may question whether or not it is desirable to carry on living. As was pointed out earlier, more requests for euthanasia arise from that desperate situation than from the ravages of physical pain. In such circumstances, however distressing they may be, the compassionate presence of those closest to the patient can become a vitally important source of comfort and aid.

CARING FOR THE CHRONICALLY ILL

In addition to help from their personal networks, people suffering from chronic illness may also receive the physical and emotional support provided by health and social care organizations. But what about those who must endure the fatigue caused by chronic illness alone at home, or those who are attended by family carers who may find that they too are in need of support?

The opening pages of this book gave a brief account of how Lindsay Clarke became the full-time carer of his wife for the five years between the first diagnosis of dementia and the day of her death. Much as they loved one another, the prolonged stress of that situation proved deeply wearing for both of them. Reflecting on that experience, he says:

There were times when I felt to be at my wit's end, driven by repetitious circumstances into impatient responses that were instantly followed by deep regret. I was also haunted by the thought that a time must come when I was no longer able to cope at all. That would certainly have happened had it not been for the help and respite provided by visits from daughters who lived far away. Those breaks allowed me to get away for a night or two to clear my head and recover composure.

More frequently, I was given the assistance of a network of friends who would come by to spend a couple of hours with my wife so that I could get out of the house, spend time in the pub with other people or visit other friends who had a compassionate understanding of the situation. I have never been a person who finds it easy to ask for help but that kindly network of willing helpers turned out to be both easier to recruit and larger than I expected. Not only did it prove beneficial – essential even – to my own sanity, it also gave my wife the pleasure of more varied company. Beyond that, it meant that I was kept in good enough shape to give her a better quality of care than might otherwise have been possible.

The support provided by relatives, friends and volunteers can make a big difference to the lives of people in need, but even simple offers to help with practical necessities can raise sensitive issues which require delicate handling. Tasks that ill people have been used to performing for themselves may carry a symbolic value intimately bound up with their identity. In offering them help, we first need to take note of what is personally important to them and find out which aspects of self-help they are prepared to relinquish. A sensitivity to their personal dignity will be sure to ask in what ways they are willing to accept help, rather than acting on assumptions about what would be helpful.

People in debilitating circumstances are undergoing involuntary changes to their lives which may radically disturb the whole pattern of their experience. Offers of help may answer such needs as assistance with shopping and other household chores, but they can also act as painful reminders of what has been lost. For example, the freedom that comes with the ability to drive a car, either for business or pleasure, is important to most people, and the offer of a lift, with its implied recognition that the person is no longer safe at the wheel, can bring a stark reminder of their deteriorating condition. With a still larger consequence, people obliged to move into a care home for the rest of their days may suffer a demoralizing shock of loss.

Such a big upheaval calls a large part of one's personal identity into question. Independence has gone. Things that were of value may have to be left behind and, because the number of care homes is limited, it might be necessary to move away from a familiar location. In such circumstances, once reliable mental maps of the surrounding environment become redundant and have to be reoriented. It is through our relationship to the people and places we know and love that we recognize ourselves, and our personal identities are reflected in both, they are rendered vulnerable by change.

Again, in such circumstances, the caring embrace and sensitive understanding of one's inner network of family and friends is of crucial importance. Such quality social contact, enriched by love, laughter and friendship, restores a sense of purpose and value to people suffering from ill health. There may be only limited ways of creating such occasions – even the visits of grandchildren may prove exhausting to the sick – but kindness and compassion can alleviate the loneliness and distress resulting from increasing weakness and fatigue.

Even small acts make a big difference. A warm letter or email from a friend instantly makes a person feel better because a number of transformative events are happening as it is read. We are touched that someone has taken the time and trouble to write to us. Biochemically, this causes an inward cascade, involving oxytocin, dopamine, serotonin and many other hormones. At the same time, our blood pressure goes down, relaxing us, so that life feels a little easier. The impact of this continues as a further shot of benevolent hormones occurs whenever we think of that friend. This might prompt the desire to ring them, or to write a reply arranging a meeting, from which further health benefits ensue. All this derives from a single, thoughtful act.

Every network will contain a number of such kindly friends, each responding in slightly different ways. One person writes an email, another uses the phone. One drops by with flowers, another offers to take us out for coffee. The benefits of such gestures can quickly accumulate as people respond. With each action taken, small or large, hearts are lifted, loads are shared, outlooks changed. The problems may remain, but such willingly offered support makes them feel less oppressive and easier to bear.

ENHANCING NETWORKS IN TIMES OF NEED

When people are suffering, it is the response of a whole network that can make the biggest difference. Twenty people offering small amounts of help will have a larger effect than the response of a single person, however well-intentioned that person may be. But there are often resistances that have to be overcome before any help is accepted at all.

A common sequence of events often occurs when we learn that someone is going through hard times. It runs along these lines: a willing helper says, 'I'm really sorry to hear about your illness. It must be very hard for you. Is there anything I can do to help?' To which, far more often than not, the answer comes, 'No thanks, we're managing fine at the moment.'

Potentially helpful social networks routinely collapse through such acts of polite refusal. When someone has offered help two or three times only to have the offers declined, they are left stuck for what to say. Next time, they might even cross the street rather than face a further rebuff. So why do people put up such barriers to the building of supportive networks and how might those barriers be overcome?

A principal resistance to accepting offers of help stems from the fear of becoming a burden to those on whom one depends. This is particularly the case with those who are accustomed to think of themselves as givers of support rather than as receivers. However, most people who willingly give support do not think of it as burdensome; rather they consider it to be a privilege. This is not difficult to understand because lending assistance or showing active care for someone who needs support makes us feel good about ourselves. It gives us the same kind of pleasurable hormonal response that happens when we receive acts of kindness.

Similarly, people in need of help will commonly insist that they don't want support from their children because they know that they are busy getting on with their own lives. But surely the decision about whether or not to give help rests with the person offering it? The resistance to accepting that help might be removed if the person refusing aid is asked how they would feel if they were to make a genuine offer of help only to have it declined.

Julian Abel recalls two examples to illustrate this point. In an outpatient discussion with an elderly couple, one of whom was likely to die of terminal cancer within a relatively short period of time, he urged them to consider their need for the support of a caring network. The next time he saw them was in an emergency admission room where they were accompanied by some of their children who said that their parents had not only refused their offers of help but would not answer the phone or open the door. 'When we looked at how that might make the children feel,' Julian says, 'it finally became obvious to the couple that they were effectively denying them the opportunity to care for their parents at the end of their lives.'

On another occasion, after giving a talk at a meeting, Julian was approached by a retired doctor who said how much he had enjoyed the talk. 'However,' he added, 'when I come to die, I would like to be put in a nursing home and be left alone. My children are busy and I don't want to bother them.' When asked why he would want to deny his children the opportunity to look after the father they loved at the end of his life, he replied, 'I hadn't thought of it that way.'

Concerns about privacy are another common reason for refusing help. Both the ill person and their resident carer may too quickly assume that an offer of help will entail an invasion of their home at a time when they are already feeling vulnerable. But such cases raise important issues of dignity and respect around the way support is given, not about the support itself. As was discussed earlier, there are many different ways of giving help, but the most successful will usually display a measure of tact and appropriate distance in the manner of their approach.

A deeply moving example of the effectiveness of an approach characterized by such respectful distance was given in a story recorded by the journalist Florence Deguen in former French newspaper *Aujourd'hui* on 5 September 2007. The article is about the work of the Gineste-Marescotti training institute, which teaches that 'miracles can be achieved with a little human kindness'. It tells the story of an 85-year-old woman called Jeanne who had to be force-fed because she had withdrawn from the world a year and a half previously by lying in her bed in a foetal position with her eyes almost always closed. One day, a trained care assistant quietly approached her saying, 'Please, Jeanne, I'm a friend,' before gently asking if she would open her eyes. No flicker of response came. When further patient attempts at coaxing met with no success, the assistant softly put a hand to Jeanne's shoulder. After a few moments, as if called back from a great distance, Jeanne opened her eyes in a vague, bewildered stare. Some time later she sat up, allowed herself to be washed and uttered her first word of assent in over a year. Eventually she even walked again and on that day she said to the assistant, 'I love you.' A film of those events is shown as part of the institute's training programme, always to moving effect.

What the story demonstrates is that establishing a correct measure of undemanding distance and acting with respect for the dignity and autonomy of the person in need of care can have profoundly important transformative effect. The assistant in Jeanne's story had been trained by the institute to respond in this way, but the same approach can be applied in everyday domestic circumstances. Checking in on friends and family can be done without any air of condescension in a manner that challenges neither their privacy nor their self-esteem. At the most basic level, a friendly telephone call simply asking someone how they are doing can make a big difference to their day and open up opportunities to give more support.

That said, non-specific offers of help can prove difficult for the receiver. Rather than simply asking, 'Is there anything I can do to help?', there is a better chance of eliciting a positive response if one identifies a particular problem with which help might be appreciated. Offers of a lift to the supermarket, or to pick up something from the shops, or to mow the lawn or walk the dog – such well-defined suggestions are more likely to be welcomed than a vague expression of a willingness to help. Some people find it easier to assent to the offer of a particular task being taken off their hands than they would asking for something specific to be done. Effective supportive networks arise as a response to real needs and those needs are identified by careful listening. Sometimes, of course, people have simply got out of the practice of responding positively when help is offered – 'I'm fine, thanks,' can become a reflex reaction – so it can help to remind them to 'Just say yes' whenever anyone asks if there is anything they can do.

There are times too when offers of support might reach out beyond the person who is ill to assist their closer network of carers. A person who loves their ill partner and wishes to do their best for them may become emotionally and physically exhausted through trying to cope alone. The demands of full-time care can push people to their limits, reaching the point where such a lonely commitment becomes unrealistic. This creates a doubly difficult situation because some aspect of the ill person's needs may not have been met and the carer is left struggling with a sense of failure. The accompanying feelings of guilt can be particularly painful when caring for someone at the end of their life. Caring is a marathon not a sprint, and the resilient support of a caring network can make all the difference between an ill person being able to remain at home and an emergency admittance to hospital.

Julian recalls the story of a colleague's mother, an elderly lady who was caring for her husband as he suffered from terminal cancer:

My colleague was at his parents' house one day, sitting in the kitchen talking to his mother, when a neighbour popped her head around the back door and said, 'Is there anything I can get you? I'm just going down the shops.' Because they had already discussed the advantages of just saying yes, his mother said, 'Yes, a pint of milk would be great, thank you,' despite the fact that she already had a fridge full of milk. When the neighbour came back, they sat down together and had a cup of tea. Not only did she enjoy the neighbour's support, both of them benefited from the social interaction.

ELECTRONIC SOURCES OF HELP

As well as forgetting how simply to say yes, we might also have lost the skill of knowing how to ask for help – perhaps because we are worried that our request will be refused, or we are overly concerned that people will consider us incapable. A practical way of getting around this problem is through the use of electronic apps, some of which are available for free.

The Jointly app is an app designed by carers for carers. Accessible through a smartphone or the internet, the app has a variety of functions including, among others, posting messages and recording a medication chart along with the names and contact details of people in the caring network with a calendar of their availability. A message might go out with a request like, 'Can anyone cook a meal on Tuesday evening as there is no one else around?' To ask a single individual such a question directly can be awkward as they might want to help but feel conflicted because they are busy at that time. But if the message goes out to 20 people, the chances are that one of them will be able to say yes. Having seen that positive reply, others will be encouraged to make offers of their own, and in this way, the sense of belonging to a team of support is strengthened and the resources of the network increased.

For some older people, using an app will not be appropriate, but a younger member of the caring network who is more familiar with electronic media may be happy to take on the role of organizer. In doing so, they will discover that running the app and seeing how people are joining in the efforts of the team can itself be a satisfying source of comfort and support.

Other potentially useful apps and social media platforms include MealTrain, GatherMyCrew, Facebook and WhatsApp, all of which can make the co-ordination of a network easier. They can also overcome the problems created by geography, as when, for instance, children live some distance from their ageing parents. With everyone co-ordinating their plans using a social-networking app, it becomes possible to check the calendar of needs and fill any gaps so that help is given by a rolling sequence of visitors, rather than everyone landing on the doorstep at the same time.

CARING FOR THE DYING

Julian tells how, when his mother was admitted to hospital with pneumonia, she was also diagnosed with leukaemia.

> *When she learned that there was no cure for her illness, nor even of lengthening her life, she made the decision that undergoing chemotherapy, with only a very small chance of it having any benefit, was not for her. While she was still in hospital, we asked her about what she wanted to do and where she would prefer to die. She said she would like to spend as much time as she could at home and then die in the hospice.*
>
> *Once we knew her wishes, we set about organizing how best to fulfil them. As is the case with many families, relationships in ours have not always been harmonious, but we put all this aside and focussed on making the most of the time remaining for my mother. During the month she was at home, people were constantly around to help. As she became less well, her inner network of close family members, including my stepfather, children, grandchildren and dear friends spent most of the time with her. Everyone took turns to keep her company and to make sure that the necessary domestic tasks were always done.*
>
> *By the time she was bedbound, the shopping, cooking and cleaning were all done by a constant flow of kindly people, which meant that those of us in her inner network could spend more time with her. After she had been at home for a couple of weeks, we re-checked with her about where she wanted to die. She said, 'I feel so comfortable and cared for at home, I would like to die here'.*
>
> *During the last weeks of my mother's life, she was surrounded by love, kindness and support. I felt that she was more content at this point in her life than at any other time I could remember. We continued to look after her at home, where she died peacefully.*

The sadness of the experience was imbued with gratitude for the way everything had happened. We were able to do the best we could for her and it worked well. The family relationships became much closer as we united in our compassionate efforts to care for her. The closeness we developed throughout that time has remained with us over the last four years. The sadness of our bereavement was shared, but so too was the sense of being uplifted by the whole experience of caring for my mother.

Compassionate networks are particularly important for those who are caring for people who are nearing the ends of their lives. They serve both a practical and an emotional purpose. Death, dying, loss and care-giving present challenges for all involved. The person with the illness may feel diminished and less valuable as a human being, and being unable to carry out simple daily tasks can lead to the loss of a sense of identity. For example, no longer being able to participate in day-to-day activities around the house, stopping driving or having to give up your job can remove important symbolic and practical roles, resulting in a sense of worthlessness. This is further complicated by having to accommodate the certainty of mortality. In these moments, the love and affection of an inner network of family and friends is particularly powerful. A sense of self-worth is restored through the kindness of others.

At the same time, the caring network benefits from similar support. When care falls on a small number of people, exhaustion is common. Dealing with the health crises that can happen towards the end of life, both physical and emotional, may be more than the resilience of smaller caring networks can manage. Dividing practical tasks between a broad range of people helps to significantly bolster this resilience. Sharing out the daily activities of shopping, cooking, cleaning and doing the garden helps enormously. A small task may be no burden at all to an individual but it can make a big difference to the main carers; each task shared is one less thing for them to do. In addition, while it goes without saying that the person with the illness should be supported and nourished through love and affection, the same is true for the caring network. Mutual support, compassion and kindness nourishes the warmth of heart of both the person doing the giving as well as the person on the receiving end. The effect is amplified when people are feeling hard-pressed through the challenges of caring while trying to accommodate the prospect of losing their life partner. Given that the majority of deaths are among the elderly, partners and spouses may well be frail themselves. Compassionate networks are not just desirable; they are vital at the end of life.

CHAPTER 8

COMPASSION IN
GENERAL PRACTICE

For obvious reasons, a visit to the doctor is often a tense affair. A long wait for an appointment or a couple of hours spent nervously waiting in a drop-in clinic may well add to the anxiety felt by a patient at this vulnerable time. We may even feel somewhat infantilized by an awareness of our dependent ignorance before an authority figure. But a consultation can be a stressful experience for the GP too. To emphasize the recurrent nature of that stress, let's consider again Dr Ann Robinson's troubling description of a typical morning's agenda in her GP surgery, as she described it in the *Guardian*, that we quoted from in chapter two. The problems that her patients presented with included depression, low self-esteem, agoraphobia, anxiety and chronic pain – none of which could be effectively treated by medication and all of which were exacerbated by social isolation.

How, one might well wonder, is a doctor to cope when faced day after day by a waiting room in which many patients are evidently suffering from something they find hard to bear yet do not present with any immediately identifiable medical condition?

Such circumstances raise the not always clear-cut question of what it means to be ill. Does the patient have a physical problem that can be sorted by medical intervention or is there a mental component to the illness? Can we in fact separate physical illness from what is happening in the mind? What about the fears and anxieties active in the patient's mind that are having a deleterious effect on their well-being but do not fit neatly into the International Classification of Diseases? And even those illnesses which can be identified as such may have a stressful social and psychological impact beyond their evident set of symptoms and signs.

The Compassionate Communities model of healthcare views illness not as an isolated incident in a person's life. Rather it is the culmination of a series of events and consequences. By the time someone presents at the surgery with a classifiable physical illness, the processes that have led up to that condition may have been at work for many years, particularly if the patient has endured prolonged stressful circumstances during that time.

Many diseases start from a background of long-term inflammation, which is in itself a response to stress. Stress can be classified as having three sources – physical, chemical and emotional – and the biochemical pathways for all three of these converge. A stress response, whether caused by single or multiple factors, results in a hormonal cascade. The chemicals released into the bloodstream alter the hormonal balance causing the secretion of steroids over prolonged periods. The loss of the normal circadian rhythm of hormone secretion has a long-term impact on the body, causing sleep disruption, weight gain and persistent inflammation, while also reducing the immune system's capacity to withstand disease. Many auto-immune diseases seen with increasing frequency over recent decades – such as thyroiditis, coeliac disease and rheumatoid arthritis – are a marker of such dysfunctional immunity. Put together, all these factors provide a further source of stress which causes and aggravates a further combination of anxiety and depression.

Chronic inflammation has a variety of consequences and plays a part in many illnesses. The widespread inflammatory impact of cigarette smoking on the body, for example, can damage blood vessels, lungs, skin, kidneys and the bladder along with other organs. Even certain types of psychotic mental illness are now thought to be caused by inflammatory, auto-immune responses. Markers can be found in the blood when we undergo such a response.

These inflammatory biochemical responses evolved as an appropriate response of the human body to short-term dangerous situations in the natural environment but they are also activated in people who suffer from such long-term mental stresses as those generated by traumatic events in childhood, difficult domestic circumstances, the pressures of a demanding job or the strains of psychiatric illness. What goes on in our mind has an impact on our health just as the chemicals released during illness affect our emotions and thoughts. In fact, mind and body are so fused that separating them is merely a conceptual convenience that bears no substantial relation to reality.

So when doctors accept that what goes on in the mind has a significant impact on bodily processes they can begin to make use of that understanding in positive ways. Such awareness will prompt the employment of comprehensive strategies designed to improve both the patient's physical welfare and their general quality of life, despite the limitations that illness may bring. Steering the body away from the generation of inflammatory chemicals and thus creating better conditions for feelings of health and well-being acts as an effective antidote to many of the problems created by stress. It can encourage greater resilience in coping with life's difficulties, improve sleep and the ability to relax, lower blood pressure and help the patient deal more positively with the other impacts the illness wreaks on both body and mind.

The challenge that this approach presents to primary healthcare teams is how to create a viable working method that integrates the physical and biochemical model of the body with the emotional and social components of the patient's overall situation. Fortunately, the recent changes made to consultation procedures at the health centre in Frome furnish a demonstrably successful example of how this essential process of integration can be implemented within the confines of a busy general practice.

REORGANIZING PRIMARY CARE

Einstein has been quoted as saying that the definition of insanity is doing the same thing over and over again and expecting a different result. The words might serve as a reminder that simply doing more of what currently happens in conventional GP surgeries will not solve the chronic problems of systematic overuse, overcrowding and rapidly increasing costs that many national health services face. Something has to give and the significant changes made by Frome Medical Practice to bring an effective Compassionate Communities programme into routine clinical care can be summarized in four main points:

- Changing the nature of clinical consultations by introducing a Compassionate Communities approach to patient care.
- Making structural changes inside the GP practice to set up efficient hubs for the identification and proactive support of people in need.

- Holding regular face-to-face team meetings to discuss individual patient care inside the practice, to gain broader multi-professional views on the management of complex cases and to solve problems that arise when working across organizational boundaries.

- Ensuring that the changes are applied in a systematic manner, designed by the people who do the work rather being forced on teams from the top down. This process comes from the Institute of Heathcare's quality improvement methodology, and is explained in more detail below.

THE COMPASSIONATE COMMUNITIES APPROACH TO HEALTHCARE

As earlier chapters have shown, one of the most important factors determining health and welfare is a lively network of good social relationships, but medical services, as currently configured, are limited in their ability to take advantage of that knowledge. When illness is strictly defined by specific categories of disease and the practice of medicine is based on the treatment of those categories, it becomes difficult to justify interventions that fall outside that system of classification. The current situation is further limited by the fact that in England appointments with GPs usually last no longer than ten minutes.

Because many illnesses present in familiar ways, they tend to elicit a well-established protocol of responses. Thus, during a conventional consultation, the doctor will ask the patient about the nature of the problem, take notes, conduct a physical examination where necessary, reach a diagnosis and come up with a management plan that employs tested treatments appropriate for that diagnosis.

If the case is more complex, then arrangements will be made for any further tests that might be needed and the patient may be referred to a specialist in the condition.

Most doctors are, of course, sensitive enough to discern when a patient is carrying additional stress and anxiety, but a ten-minute session amid a busy schedule of urgent priorities allows little time for enquiry into the person's social circumstances. Even if such issues were explored it's probable that the doctor would have little more to offer than a few carefully chosen words of sympathy.

By contrast, in a well-established culture of Compassionate Communities, such as that found in Frome, the process of clinical consultation is approached with broader perspectives and different expectations in mind. The conventional medical model, which focuses mostly on physical and chemical factors, is expanded to include exploration of any relevant psychological and social causes of stress. The available resources of the surrounding social environment are then brought into consideration to open up wider possibilities for treatment than those offered by an exclusively pharmaceutical response.

In the context of the Compassionate Communities approach to primary care, a doctor confronted by patients for whom medical expertise alone is not sufficient will have immediate access to a directory of services displaying the wide range of locally available resources which might help to answer the need for support, advice, assistance and companionship in a wide variety of circumstances.

With those resources in mind, the doctor will question patients about their overall situation, prompting pause for thought about the ways in which their personal circumstances might be contributing to their illness. Whether the patients are troubled by problems at home or in their work relationships, by loneliness or poor eating habits, or any of the other stressful difficulties encountered in modern life, referring them to local sources of help to address those issues can improve both their health and their general morale.

The model of the Compassionate Frome project has radically improved both the nature of the conversation between doctor and patient and the interaction between the medical practice and the people of the town. Such changes are made much easier if the expectations that patients bring to the consultation include a willingness to think imaginatively about how the habitual course of their lives might be having a negative impact on their health and welfare and how it might be enhanced. But in both personal and social terms, for both medical professionals and the people they serve, the benefits yielded by close creative liaison between primary care and the wider structure of a Compassionate Community can be immense.

Dr Helen Kingston recalls a patient who came to see her because she had been told to go to the medical practice and ask for renewal of the prescription for the medication she had been taking for depression following her move to the town. When Helen asked why she needed the medication, it emerged that the patient had recently moved from a neighbouring town after violence within her family. She was now precariously sofa surfing. She came asking for more medication for her depression but desperately wanted help to extricate herself from her itinerant position and rebuild her life.

Confronted by such circumstances, the conventional medical model would probably have renewed the prescription and then referred the patient to social services, at which point it might have taken weeks to arrange the help with housing that was clearly needed. The Compassionate Communities model offered a different approach, in which the next step was to see what was immediately available in the way of help and support for the patient. Having identified the patient's needs, Helen consulted the Health Connections Mendip directory, clicking on housing and homelessness. The options immediately revealed ranged from support for those who had suffered domestic abuse and support with accommodation information including advice for rough sleepers to a rough sleeper helpline and housing options with Mendip District Council. Another click opened the section on poverty/finance/grants for immediate problems related to homelessness and information on the availability of free meals and other sources of practical help. Beyond those immediately relevant sources of information lay other, more general resources, such as attending a talking café where a health connector could offer more direct advice. A further wide range of helpful information is available under the various mental health headings.

The ability to immediately access a list of local resources relevant to the patient's circumstances demonstrates how, even in the context of a ten-minute appointment, the GP can give any necessary attention to symptoms and signs of illness and then direct the conversation to the readily available support of a Compassionate Community. The doctor and patient can explore possibilities together and discuss what might prove most helpful among the variety of options on display. Having been given this kind of help to make informed choices, the patient can then take away a print-out of relevant material to follow up for themself.

Of course, not every problem can be discussed and solved in a single consultation, but once this community-based approach has equipped patients to begin to think differently, and more creatively, in relation to their condition, they can be encouraged to use the information to plan a line of action for its improvement. A further appointment, a week later perhaps, would discuss progress on whatever was achieved in the first consultation and explore ways to build on it. Such a scenario – connecting health issues to other underlying problems and exploring feasible means to act on them – offers more hope for improving a patient's life than merely prescribing medication.

As Helen says, 'It may seem to many GPs that taking this approach is likely to be more time consuming. However, I have found that it actually saves time: partly because I can address what is important to the patient and partly because it can save large amounts of time investigating something which is not the main problem.' Because doctors are motivated by a compassionate desire to help people, if they are given the right tools, they will provide the best help they can.

The example given above also gives an indication of how patients' expectations of the consultation process might be changed. The normal assumption is that the job of a doctor is to treat illness, not to engage with the wider issues and circumstances of the patient's life. So the patient turns up seeking a medical cure (for depression in this case) and expects that to be the topic of brief conversation. From this patient's point of view, it might have initially felt a lot easier simply to ask for medication than to talk about recent imprisonment, homelessness and the associated feelings of vulnerability. But for many patients, having the doctor help them plan what might be done to improve their overall situation on more than just a purely medical level is far more motivating than being handed some pills. Part of the Compassionate Communities approach is to help individuals recognize their own strengths and support networks. This is found through enquiring about what matters most to them, what has worked well and what has made a positive difference in the past. The project enables different conversations. Knowing that there are resources to offer makes those conversations easier, as asking what the individual already has and is doing to strengthen their own support is safe. If they cannot think of anything, the clinician has something to offer from the service directory, knowing that a wide variety of resources can be found there. This creates the freedom to explore the non-medical aspects with confidence. Making some suggestions and providing information can be successful when it helps an individual to open a conversation with their own existing support network and to recognize how much others already value them.

It's possible, of course, that some patients will lack either the energy or the desire to take advantage of the support on offer in the community. Even a short illness can drain one's energy, while prolonged illness often leads to chronic fatigue, loss of social function and associated depression. All these factors may have a bearing on the patient's condition. Tactful questioning by the doctor can open up issues that would otherwise be missed or ignored, even though they might be critical to the proper management of the patient's illness and the prevention of longer-term health problems or undue stress being placed on the patient's carer, which could eventually lead to burn-out.

It's also possible that issues of low self-esteem and lack of self-confidence might impede the patient's motivation to take up offers of community support. In that case, reliance on the service directory alone would not be enough and the doctor can ask the patient if they would like to see someone who could help them to deal more effectively with the problems that are troubling them. The role of the health connector – with their training in motivational interviewing – then proves invaluable. As was previously discussed, they know what is going on in the community and how to access appropriate support. This means that they can help the patient more clearly identify the nature and source of the problems and then find the kind of advice and support that will give them the tools and the confidence to improve their situation.

Dr Helen Kingston explains below how somebody may be suffering from a variety of problems which are not resolved using therapeutics alone:

Somebody might come in talking about their back problems and diabetes but then very quickly the conversation moves on to family dynamics. Their mood and the uncertainty that they are facing are the real issues for them. There are not necessarily medical solutions to their long-term problems. Referring them to a health connector begins the process of learning to live better with their problems rather than thinking that there is a medical fix.

Helen recalls the case of a woman who presented with headaches and back pains and a combination of depression and anxiety:

A daily battle with her physical symptoms along with difficult life circumstances was exhausting and demoralizing. Rather than putting her on more and more medication it was better to listen and understand her situation. She very much wanted to break her cycle of exhaustion and chronic pain and was open to different approaches. She went to see a health connector who helped her focus on her priorities. She decided to join a pain management programme and, afterwards, despite still coping with a divorce and looking after a young family, she set up a small business making a variety of items and selling them. As well as enjoying doing this and getting a lot of satisfaction from her talents, it was her way of managing her life. Her symptoms got better because she was able to channel some of her efforts into something creatively satisfying rather than focusing on what her problems were. Having

*come through a difficult time she was more aware of the support
she had around her. She used to come in with a long list of what
needed fixing but this changed to what her priorities were. I don't
see her as often now. She has the tools necessary to deal with the
next problem that may hit her. She was resourceful and knew best
her own way out of a difficult situation. She has shown herself
that she has the network around her and the skills to apply to any
future problems.*

This illustrates the importance of the role of the health
connector in the compassionate approach to general practice.
Using motivational interviewing techniques, a health connector
will ask questions that bring to the surface what really matters
most to the patient and then they can set goals together and
formulate a plan. This process of goal setting differs from that
of care planning, which is a medical process in which patients
are asked to make choices about situations they would prefer to
avoid. This might, for example, include plans to avoid hospital
admission, heroic medical interventions or resuscitation. By
contrast, goal setting is about improving well-being and a positive
way of engaging with matters important to the patient's life – such
as overcoming the emotional difficulties of loneliness or the grief
of bereavement, or the problems raised by practical issues such as
those of housing and employment.

If confidence to go out into the community or to join a new group
is low, then the health connector might suggest they accompany
the patient on the first occasion. Help would also be given with
practical considerations, such as the need for a lift from a volunteer
transport scheme. If no such scheme exists, the health connector
will ask community developers to start one.

STRUCTURAL CHANGES INSIDE
GENERAL PRACTICE

The adoption of a Compassionate Communities model involves more than changes to the nature of the consultation process. Each GP surgery will need to work out how best to build its requirements into the routine of daily work. Methods of identifying patients in need of the kind of support it offers and then tracking their progress will have to be put in place, and this will require a shift in the mindset of both practice workers and patients.

Not all patients who make contact with the primary care team may need to see a doctor to access appropriate help and support. When surgery receptionists who have been trained as community connectors answer patients' calls and are told the nature of the problem, they may recognize an opportunity to save valuable appointment time by directly referring callers to helpful resources in the services directory.

As we saw in the previous chapter, the role of the community connector is vital to the practical development of an actively compassionate pattern of social life within a community. The Frome model demonstrates that anyone who wishes to be involved can train in a couple of hours to become an effective community connector, and the example just given illustrates how the provision of such training can make the practice's initial diagnosis of a patient's needs more efficient. The key function of the role is to help people familiarize themselves with, and navigate their way through, relevant information about the many kinds of support that are available within the community. That helpful service can be delivered by every trained member of staff within a medical practice. Thus, reception at the front desk of Frome Medical Practice is staffed by navigators who know how to direct people towards the kind of support they most urgently need, whether that is an appointment with a doctor or another resource listed in the service directory.

If a medical practice is to take full advantage of the resources offered by the Compassionate Communities approach, it will need to consider what specific functions that approach will serve and how best they can be managed from a central hub. At a minimum, such a hub will consist of trained administrative staff who are able to identify patients in need of assistance, establish and maintain contact with them, and refer them to health connectors as necessary. When requested, they will also make arrangements for oversight by the multi-disciplinary team, made up of doctors, nurses, physiotherapists and other health and social care professionals, including the health connectors. Where relevant, this team also liaises with hospitals to enable a patient's swift and effective discharge, making sure that everything is in place for someone to be looked after safely at home. All of this requires careful planning and investment.

IDENTIFICATION OF THOSE IN NEED OF SUPPORT

In Frome, practical experience has shown that a good time to contact someone is after discharge from hospital. Even when the hospital treatment has gone well, the experience can be depersonalizing and traumatic, and most people are keen not to revisit hospital if it can be avoided. At that critical moment they are usually ready to consider other ways in which to address their health issues.

Dr Helen Kingston recalls the case of a patient admitted to hospital with a possible vascular problem that fortunately turned out not to be serious.

But the patient lived on her own and the hospital admission was a frightening experience for her. It shook her confidence. That was an opportunity to look at the bigger uncertainty in her life and to consider the things that were most important to her. It became easier to have a conversation about vulnerability and living on her own. She had children living locally who rallied around as a consequence of our conversation. Bringing them together didn't just meet her physical needs; she had a great supportive network around her and was able to re-orientate her support.

A phone call after discharge from hospital will begin that process. Certain routine medical and nursing issues will be checked – is there a need for blood tests, has a medication regime changed, should follow-up appointments be made? But it is equally important to ask about the patient's domestic and social circumstances. Is additional support needed? How is the main carer managing? Who else is around to help out? What limitations are patient and carer facing as a consequence of the illness or the recovery process?

Such questions extend beyond purely medical and nursing issues, and so when ancillary healthcare staff first start to ask them they may struggle somewhat. They may not even consider the issues to be relevant. But as Julianne Holt-Lunstad's paper on the link between social relationships and mortality has shown, they can be quite as important as matters of medical procedure.

Jo Trickett, who has a background of experience in looking after people with chronic health conditions in hospital, joined Frome Medical Practice in 1999 and is the practice nurse who has developed the process of ringing patients after their discharge from hospital. Describing the skills and sensitivity needed in calling people in those often uncertain circumstances, she says:

I ask open but specific questions, such as who is around you at home, have you managed to get to the shops, is there food, have you been able to get up the stairs? These are basic things we often take for granted but they are things people may not be able to do when they are struggling. This can open and create a further conversation. I listen for non-verbal clues on the phone, listening to who is in the background. You hear the sigh, the gasps or the husband moaning in the background! I recently spoke with an elderly lady who had been admitted to hospital with abdominal pain caused by the medication she was taking. Over a period of five weeks she had become increasingly housebound, having been independent and driving beforehand. She went home isolated and unsure what life was going to hold for her. She was really struggling to come to terms with where her life was going. She had neighbours who were out at work and a son who lives far away. I referred her to the health connectors who could support her. She previously went to groups and clubs and they could help her get back into her community. When I suggested it, she said, 'That would be lovely, but I can't drive.' So we can find a solution to that, with befrienders and volunteer drivers. You could almost feel the weight being lifted from her mind.

It is important not to forget the family and carers that surround the patient. I sometimes say, 'Can I have a chat with your wife or your husband? How are they getting on?' Sometimes I don't have much to do with the patient because it's all been done, but I can put the spouse in contact with the health connectors so that they can get some support. Connection with other carers can make a big difference.

There are a number of reasons why it's a good idea to contact the majority of people discharged from hospital. If someone has undergone a hip replacement, it might mean they are suffering from the longer-term consequences of aging. If they live alone and their mobility is poor, how do they manage the practical tasks of life? Is loneliness a problem? Does an elderly partner need support? Such conversations can develop quite naturally in a way that makes it easier to offer help. As Jo demonstrates, the key is for the person who is making contact to be alert to the occurrence of these kinds of problems and listen out for indicators that something else might be a problem beyond the immediate health considerations.

If the patient doesn't want immediate support, they may still be interested in seeing a health connector with a view to longer-term goal-setting and getting back out into the community. The health connector will visit patients who are housebound to make sure they are not excluded from the resources available. For the same reason, if there are patients for whom English is not their first language, the practice should arrange for leaders from within their own cultural groups to visit them so that they are not left isolated because of their ethnicity.

TEAM MEETINGS

The problems faced by patients range from the simple to the very complex and managing difficult diseases within complicated social situations might take more input than can be given by a single doctor working alone. In such cases, multi-disciplinary team meetings can bring together a range of skilled professionals.

In addition to GPs, these meetings might involve district nurses, social workers, specialists in care of the elderly, physiotherapists, discharge liaison nurses from the local hospital and others as deemed appropriate.

An important new initiative in Frome has been the inclusion of community development workers – a health connector for example – as part of the clinical team in multi-disciplinary meetings. A health connector can provide valuable input to group discussions aimed at looking for solutions to what may be a multiplicity of problems, and sometimes a whole new dimension of thought about the management of a patient's general welfare. Issues and possible solutions that might not usually occur to a GP are now taken into consideration. As a result, there have been significant changes in customary assumptions and patterns of behaviour.

For example, should it emerge that the patient under discussion is suffering from loneliness, and the health connector is able to go away and help the patient to enhance personal networks or to make good use of community resources, they may then be able to report back at a subsequent meeting with a moving story about the successful resolution of difficult problems, which inspires the doctor in charge of the case to use that pathway again when a similar situation arises.

Helen Kingston and Jenny Hartnoll recall many examples of how sharing such success stories has reshaped and invigorated the work of team members, including doctors, nurses and medical students, who have been inspired and encouraged by the life-changing effects that linking a patient to community resources can bring about. After completing her placement in Frome, one final-year medical student sent Jenny the following feedback about her experience of a talking café:

I had such a warm welcome from everyone at the café and was made to feel like one of the group immediately. It was lovely speaking to everyone and learning about what the café does and what it means to people. I was taken aback at how busy the café was and the variety of activities that were going on. It felt like I had walked into a vibrant little community right there, with everyone knowing each other and catching up. The talking café clearly means so much to the people who go along.

I spoke to people who use the café for social company, those who used it as a way of making new friends when they moved into the area, as well as people who had been coming to the café for four years and those who like me had come for the first time. Everyone was polite and friendly and truly interested in who I was and what I was doing there. It was really interesting to see how close-knit the group was and yet still so friendly and welcoming to newcomers.

I just wanted to say thank you so much for letting me come along, it's truly been an invaluable morning. These cafés clearly offer so much more to the people who use them than a 10-minute trip to the doctor. Having even just a couple of hours of positivity a week, something to look forward to, to distract from health problems or negativity, can really make such a difference in people's lives and it is something that needs to be encouraged more. I'll be sure to remember this morning as I continue throughout my career and will always remember the services you provide and recommend these to people when I can.

THE USE OF QUALITY IMPROVEMENT METHODOLOGY FOR CHANGE

Whether or not such structural changes to a general practice prove successful depends to a considerable extent on the way in which they are introduced. The method by which change is made is as important as the change itself and will be integral to its nature. For this reason, in both the introduction of the Frome model and the later roll-out across other healthcare systems, the process has been managed by using the Institute of Healthcare Quality Improvement Methodology because its key features are relevant to, and consistent with, the principles underpinning the development of Compassionate Communities. Briefly put, quality improvement is a method of delivering safe change which is designed by the people who do the work rather than by outside experts and requires that any changes be thoroughly tested before they are widely implemented. This approach is based on the fundamental assumption that those who are most directly involved care about the quality of their work and are rich in experience, resources and inventiveness. So it begins by discussing with those who do the work the nature of the problem that needs resolving and consulting them about possible solutions.

A dominant feature of the recent history of healthcare in the UK has been the top-down management of structural change. This has created enormous problems and wasted millions of pounds. As is now glaringly evident, the consequences of an approach that paid little consultative regard to the skills, knowledge and experience of those whose lives and work would be most affected by the changes have proved as disruptive as they were predictable.

In an engaging TED talk, 'Want to Help Someone? Shut Up and Listen!', the social entrepreneur Ernesto Sirolli tells a pertinent story of the wastefully inefficient consequences of taking a different, top-down approach to introducing changes. In the 1970s, while working as a motivated young man trying to help farmers in the Zambezi Valley to increase their crop yield, he joined an aid organization that was teaching farmers to grow tomatoes and courgettes. Given the plentiful sunlight and fertile soil in the region, the scheme proved immediately successful with the vegetables growing to an enormous size. Everything went well until one night a herd of hippos came out of the river and ate the whole crop. The next day the aid workers demanded to know why the farmers hadn't told them about the hippos. The farmers replied, 'Because you did not ask us.' Sirolli's wry comment on this disaster was, 'At least we fed the hippos. Many such schemes did not produce anything.'

Partly as a result of this dispiriting experience, Sirolli started a community development institute in 1985. On its website, the Sirolli Institute describes itself as an advocate for a civic economy: 'A model of development that supports the creation of wealth from within your community by nurturing the intelligence and resourcefulness of your people.' This description matches the principles of participatory community development as the means by which communities decide for themselves what their problems are and how they wish to go about resolving them.

If the same process of empowering the community to decide what they need and what will work as is central to Participatory Community Development is applied to workplaces, then the people who actually do the work, and therefore have a direct experience-based understanding of what constitutes the most efficient modes of practice, would be the arbiters of appropriate structural change.

When major initiatives are designed and imposed from above without adequate consultation, they often require additional paperwork to ensure that the changes are implemented. Then, progressively over time, each new change breeds more paperwork. The situation can be further complicated by a failure to consider how much time it takes to complete each piece of paperwork. If that measurement was made before the launch of an initiative, it would accurately predict its impracticality. To make matters worse, while an individual change might make good sense on its own terms, once it gets entangled in the history of other changes, its impacts can be disastrous.

As it is, in some hospital wards where the process of change management has been badly conducted, the situation has deteriorated to the point where nurses now spend 75 per cent of their time completing paperwork and only 25 per cent on direct patient contact. Placed under pressure by management which has an investment in enforcing the changes, the staff reluctantly do what has become an onerous duty even though they know it is wasteful of their valuable time. Those who raise objections are accused of being difficult or resistant and, in consequence, mistrust of any new changes in healthcare now prevails across wards where much of management has become synonymous with forcing people to operate systems that they know are inefficient. Quality Improvement Methodology is a far more productive way to implement change.

The second essential aspect of Quality Improvement Methodology is its demand for the thorough testing of changes before they are implemented. This is best done out in the real world through a series of testing cycles which can be quick and effective. Progressive cycles of change allow for the people who do the work to make adjustments in small, limited steps of continuous improvement. Only when sound working knowledge of the effectiveness of the proposed change is established can it then be more widely introduced.

Again, the basic assumptions of this methodology are threefold: that skilled people are competent rather than feckless; that respect should be given to their experience and that management will trust that the people who do the work are best placed to know what will work best. Granted those determining principles, relevant input from everyone involved is welcome.

Quality Improvement Methodology also insists on the building of safe, reliable systems, which is, of course, a primary requirement of all aspects of medical practice. The procedures of the aircraft industry provide a good example of what this means. Modern aircraft have as many as four million parts and each of these must work reliably for the aeroplane to perform its critical functions of taking off, staying in the air and landing safely. If a number of parts fail at the same time the aeroplane may crash, so the design of each part has to be tested in the real world and adapted until it can be trusted. The same is true in the practice of medicine. If the whole system is to work well, each component must reliably play its part.

This presiding principle is directly applicable to the employment of the Compassionate Communities approach inside general practice. Not only must the changes be designed by the people who do the work, they must be applied reliably across the whole practice. If the principles are applied to some patients and not to others, then some people will miss out on the benefits, diminishing the overall effectiveness of the programme.

The consequences of a failure to make a system comprehensive enough are illustrated by the limitations of Social Prescribing, a recently fashionable form of healthcare provision in the United Kingdom. Under that scheme, a GP who encounters a patient with problems such as extreme loneliness, which are social rather than medical, will refer them to a service that links them to some form of group activity where they can meet new people and form friendships. This sounds much like an aspect of the Compassionate Communities model. However, there are significant gaps in Social Prescribing schemes. The options offered to the patient may not suit them, and if the scheme lacks a community development arm, any gaps that become apparent will not be recognized and dealt with by putting relevant resources into place.

Jenny Hartnoll developed the talking cafés as part of the Frome model in direct response to the stated needs of people who said that they simply wanted to go to a place where they could talk to others rather than engage in a specific activity. Those conversations at the café have often highlighted other needs which could then be met.

Further problems with Social Prescribing schemes arise if the patient is unable to get out of their home because of mobility issues or is reluctant to do so because of a lack of confidence. This means that people who may be chronically unwell are excluded from the advantages of the scheme. A further weakness stems from the fact that such schemes often fail to help people to enhance their personal supportive networks as described in previous chapters.

Many good things may happen under the provision of Social Prescribing schemes, but there is a question about the overall reliability of the system. The scheme requires investment, but if too many people are excluded because they fall through the gaps without being picked up and supported, then it will not show the significant outcomes that have been demonstrated by the Frome approach to health and welfare. In an austerity economy, any scheme that fails to show the financial gains needed for long-term development is at risk of seeing its funding withdrawn with the consequential loss of all its good work.

The same principle of systems reliability has to be applied when starting a new Compassionate Communities programme of change inside a GP practice. If there are ten GPs in a practice and only five adopt that approach, then half the patients who could have benefited will be missed out. To avoid the gaps that occur in Social Prescribing schemes, the approach must be employed across the entire practice and integrated with the whole pattern of community resources.

THE THERAPEUTIC RELATIONSHIP

Both from a symbolic perspective and that of practical reality, doctors have a vitally important role in modern life. People turn to them at their most vulnerable times, whether their plight is caused by physical or mental illness. It's obvious enough that going to visit a kind, warm-hearted doctor whom we feel to be genuinely concerned for our welfare is a very different experience from consulting an efficient but emotionally distant member of the medical profession. A compassionate therapeutic relationship might be considered no more than a congenial add-on to clinical care rather than a significant contribution to the effectiveness of the treatment, but there is strong evidence that the manner in which care is delivered is itself important to the healing process and to the development of well-being.

In medical practice, double-blind, placebo-controlled trials are the standard way of determining the effectiveness of a drug. Neither doctor nor patient knows whether the drug administered is real or a placebo. Examination of the results for both groups should determine which is more effective. If the placebo, which has no active ingredients, produces the same result as the active drug, this shows that the drug is not effective.

The Compassionate Communities model, however, has shown that, in many cases, the therapeutic relationship can be more effective than the drugs being prescribed. These findings throw into question the current basis on which drugs are tested. It suggests that the practice of medicine amounts to rather more than the application of science: the quality of human relationships also has to be taken into account.

This may seem a matter of common sense to anyone in need of medical care, but for those who have put their trust solely in the scientific practice of medicine it can be a hard pill to swallow. Out of the best motivation, such doctors dedicate their lives to acquiring as much knowledge and skill as they can to limit the suffering caused by disease. They work extremely hard, sometimes to the detriment of their own work/life balance, and there can be no doubting the sincerity of their desire to relieve human pain and distress. However, the success of the Frome model of care points to the need for rather more than an exclusively scientific approach to the practice of medicine.

Between the sixteenth and twentieth centuries, scientific thought progressed through experiments based on first principles of objectivity and replicability. The volume of a glass of water can be measured to a high degree of accuracy in that way, but emotions are not so convenient. They contain no measurable substance, cannot be contained and are difficult to define. Those factors disqualified them from scientific examination, so they were ignored and left out of count. This cultural blind spot led to an increasing mistrust of emotion. But, as we have seen, emotions are vital elements in our health and well-being, and the placebo effect, which accounts for the fact that people can get better even when receiving medication which has no active ingredients, is sometimes seen by health scientists as a source of irritation which confuses scientific trials.

That might be the case if there was a way to measure the precise impact of each active ingredient in medication. What we now know is that, whether or not the medication has active ingredients, a compassionate therapeutic relationship between doctor and patient is an important factor in the healing process. Because the quality of that interaction is defined by the particular nature of the relationship between the two people involved, it cannot, of course, be standardized in the form of a clinical trial. But these days, the presence of socializing emotions can be measured and directly correlated to health. The hormones which are their messengers can be studied and calibrated, and their impact on biochemical and physical markers of disease can be observed – inwardly through metabolic pathways, high blood pressure and stress hormone production, and outwardly through significant aspects of social behaviour.

The development of this knowledge has important consequences for the proper evaluation of health and well-being. Furthermore, results observable in the Frome model strongly suggest that the warm contact between a patient and a doctor well-equipped with knowledge of available supportive resources in the surrounding community can have more benefits than the standard process of simply prescribing medication.

The reduction in emergency admissions to hospital in Frome has been important to the evolution of medical practice because it provides substantial evidence that the application of compassionate values in an integrated relationship between sound medical care and a lively pattern of community activity has measurably positive outcomes. Far from being an irritant, this form of placebo effect is an inexpensive, advantageous and salutary boon.

This means that such an approach should now be viewed as more than just a 'nice idea': it is an essential component of good medical care. If we go to see the doctor and are not treated in a compassionate manner which takes the relevant circumstances of our lives and relationships into proper account as part of the management of our illness, then the doctor is at fault. We are being denied that which is most beneficial to our health and welfare.

Medicine is a uniquely valuable human resource. That anyone who is unwell should be seen by a healthcare team is deemed to be so important to a decent life that it is included in the 1948 Universal Declaration of Human Rights. Article 25 states, 'We all have the right to enough food, clothing, housing and healthcare for ourselves and our families.'

In the United Kingdom, this is provided free of charge at the point of access, which means that it is possible to see a doctor or go to hospital without having to pay anything. Poor people are not excluded. The law governing this provision of care is in itself an embodiment of the principles of compassion and equity. Yet, as an extension of those humane principles, not only the medical needs of people but also the relevant circumstances of their lives should be taken into account. Healthcare professionals are best placed to address both needs.

The Frome model has demonstrated how such compassionate attention can be transformative in the context of both healthcare and social welfare, and the measurable success of the way in which it takes those factors into account offers a working example of a comprehensive approach which can be applied with beneficial effects by health services further afield, at home and abroad.

Of course, it is essential that the highest quality of skilled medical attention should be given, but a system fixated on targets is likely to miss the point that the quality of the kindness and compassion with which clinical treatment is administered is itself as important as that of the technical expertise. To ignore these findings and not act on them would be a failure to provide the best currently available form of care for vulnerable people.

CHAPTER 9

THE WIDER REACH OF COMPASSIONATE ACTION

A compassionate city is an uncomfortable city! A city that is uncomfortable when anyone is homeless and hungry. Uncomfortable if every child isn't loved and given rich opportunities to grow and thrive. Uncomfortable when as a community we don't treat our neighbours as we would wish to be treated.

Karen Armstrong, founder of the global movement
Charter for Compassion

The most important lesson to be drawn from what has been accomplished in Frome is that effectively applied compassion has transformative power. The community of Frome achieved such remarkable outcomes through the whole population supporting each other. This was a combined effort from the people of Frome, Health Connections Mendip, Frome Medical Practice and the independent council. That being the case, the success of the Healthcare Mendip project in Frome raises questions about the ways in which other aspects of our civic life are currently structured and about whether the underlying values and principles of Compassionate Communities might not have a similarly transformative effect across a wider social horizon.

What might be gained, for instance, through a further-reaching combined and integrated Compassionate Communities programme that takes into account our familial and friendship networks to transform the life of our neighbourhoods? How might implementation of its underlying values enhance our educational institutions, our workplaces, our system of local government, our churches, mosques and temples? Might such a groundswell of change, driven by local knowledge and lived experience, bring effective influence to bear on politicians and the way that decisions which affect our lives are made? And, rather than remaining complicit with the corrosive despair inflicted by economic austerity and social deterioration, might not a general application of the fundamental value of compassion encourage us to conceive ways of providing a better future for our children through more responsibly committed concern for the natural environment on which all our lives depend? In a time increasingly aware of the disastrous consequences of disregard for the natural order, such efforts would work for the immediate benefit, and perhaps even for the decent survival, of the world at large.

To proceed from an account of the success enjoyed by a single local project in changing the way one area of human concern is managed in a relatively small town to a wider demand for radically creative activity such as is implicit in the questions raised above, may seem disproportionately ambitious. Yet the need for change is urgently felt in many areas of our lives, and the fundamental value that could drive and guide such change – compassion – is one to which we all have access. It's also one of which, sooner or later, we all have need.

Two ideas are of particular significance here. Firstly, it's important to emphasize that the support that people give to each other is not just a matter of public duty or of ethical responsibility to care, it's also cause for celebration – a recognition that there can be joy in the giving and receiving of help.

Secondly, though the Compassionate Frome model arose out of a need to meet particular issues of health, it recognized that life's testing moments can include many other forms of trouble and distress, and it is in response to such moments of moral discomfort that active care conducted in a compassionate spirit can have a significant impact. For a more specific consideration of how this might be done, the rest of this book will examine ways in which the values and principles of Compassionate Communities can be adapted to bring about the creation of a more humane and fruitfully productive pattern of social and civic life.

COMPASSION IN EDUCATION

Findings from a survey published by the Office of National Statistics in 2017 revealed the disturbing fact that one in eight children between the ages of 5 and 19 in England was suffering from psychological distress. The rates recorded in 17 to 19-year-olds were still higher, reaching 16.9 per cent, and this worrying situation has continued to deteriorate.

In 2018, a survey of the mental and emotional distress suffered by children in the British schooling system was published by the teenage mental health charity stem4. It found that, during the course of the previous year, almost four out of five (78 per cent) of the 300 teachers responding to the survey claimed to have seen a pupil dealing with difficult mental health problems. High levels of anxiety featured prominently among the reported cases, but they also included widespread depression, eating disorders, drug addiction and self-harm. Of those children whose suffering had been of concern to the teachers, 14 per cent had confessed to suicidal thoughts or shown signs of potentially suicidal behaviour. Meanwhile, barely half of all the children involved in the survey had been given access to treatment by the NHS child and adolescent mental health services (CAMHS), even though their teachers believed that such treatment was urgently needed.

Many parents are well aware of the levels of anxiety experienced by small children preparing for their SATs exams (Standard Assessment Tests) at the end of year two. Such nervous stress can continue to haunt them as they progress from level to level throughout their educational careers. Teachers (whose efficiency is being indirectly measured by the tests) are equally aware of the harm that such anxiety can do.

Commenting on the findings of the stem4 survey, a consultant clinical psychologist, Dr Nihara Krause, said, 'Schools face huge challenges in dealing with mental issues in their students, and teachers are on the front line. They witness first-hand the devastating impact of such pressures as exam anxiety, bullying and family problems. The consequences of these problems are serious, often life-threatening, and teachers are desperate to help.' Yet schools are finding it increasingly difficult to provide preventative and other specialist services that such stressful circumstances demand.

Nor is it only the pupils who are struggling. A poll of teachers published by the National Education Union (NEU) in 2019 found that a fifth of teachers, many of them recently trained, plan to leave the profession in the next two years. Two-fifths of teachers and support staff also hope to leave in the next five years because they claim that the demands of the accountability regime and the other workload pressures are 'out of control'. One of the responding teachers complained that, 'My job is no longer about children. It's just a 60-hour week with pressure to push children's achievement data through.' Others claimed that the stress of increased class sizes, a growing assessment workload and a lack of support staff had damaging effects on their personal work/life balance, and that 'a job in education is not conducive to family life.'

Responding to the education secretary's plans to prevent the accelerating flight of experienced teachers from the classroom, Kevin Courtney, the joint general secretary of the NEU said that, 'So long as the main drivers of a performance-based system are still in place, schools will continue to be in the grip of a culture of fear, over-regulation and a lack of trust. We need drastic action and a major rethink from government if we are to stop the haemorrhaging of good teachers from the profession.'

In addition to those stresses, a survey of 5,000 teachers conducted by the NASUWT teacher's union in 2019 found that one in four of them experienced some form of violence every week; nine out of ten were subjected to verbal abuse and 46 per cent had been physically threatened. Not all schools are, of course, facing such severe conditions, and the sources of those problems can be traced outside the schools to such factors as poor parenting skills (often aggravated by financial poverty), familial breakdown and the general loss of a sound moral compass in society at large. One alarming consequence of all those factors has been the recent increase in knife crime, which is often committed by young people who have been excluded from school.

In all these areas, the creation of a widespread culture of Compassionate Communities would be beneficial in its effects. The introduction of such benevolent measures in schools would certainly improve the quality of life for pupils and teachers alike.

One can fairly assume that, as far as most teachers are concerned, the desire to become a teacher at all indicates a reasonably high level of moral commitment and a degree of care for the welfare of others. Yet something seems to have gone badly wrong with the professional structures within which they work, and with the expectations of an education system that is now substantially driven by impersonal modes of targeting, standardization and productivity akin to those which typically drive industrial processes. It seems to have become an oppressive system which too many young teachers – who may once have hoped to be role models of intelligence, enthusiasm and creativity to their pupils – now flee rather than risk a burnt-out future of cynicism and disillusionment such as is increasingly found in the staff rooms of our schools and colleges.

Yet things don't have to be this way. For many years, the distinguished educational thinker Sir Ken Robinson has been arguing for a system of education that prioritizes the distinctive individuality of each pupil rather than the standardizing factors, such as age, which they have in common. He champions a pedagogy that looks for ways to enhance children's enthusiasm for learning, to explore both their personal creativity and their pleasure in collaboration, to encourage curiosity and the ability to question and thereby stimulate the sense of wonder. Should such a liberating approach sound impractical as a general curriculum, he points to what has already been achieved by the system of education in Finland, a country that produces some of the best outcomes in Europe.

In describing its country's vision for its schools, the Finnish National Board of Education places the focus on learning rather than testing, so there are no national tests for basic education. Teaching is regarded as a high-status profession in Finland and, having been allowed the discretion to design their own curriculum, teachers are trusted with the responsibility of assessing performance on the basis of its objectives. This liberated system of schooling produces an internationally recognized high standard of results in maths, science and reading as well as across a broad and diverse curriculum of study.

In a characteristically witty TED talk titled 'How to Escape Education's Death Valley', Ken Robinson tells of a group of teachers who visited Finland from the USA where, at enormous economic costs to the country, 60 per cent of the students drop out of high school. When Finnish teachers were asked how they cope with the drop-out problem, they looked at one another somewhat bemused and said they had no experience of it.

It seems unlikely that those teachers have much of a problem with school exclusion either. The young people of Finland are clearly thriving in a happier climate of schooling than currently exists in England where, for economic purposes, a highly politicized strategy of top-down management has developed an impersonal national curriculum of study. As a dominant aspect of its culture of conformity, teachers and pupils alike are subjected to a competitive and highly reductive battery of tests and inspections.

As Ken Robinson points out, such a system is not only out of phase with the natural diversity, curiosity and creativity of human beings, it is also likely to stifle them, and is therefore fated to create the kind of problems that currently bedevil it. Such a delivery system of knowledge and testing is fundamentally opposed to the spirit of compassionate imagination to which Albert Einstein referred when he insisted that, 'Imagination is more important than knowledge. For knowledge is limited, whereas imagination embraces the entire world, stimulating progress, giving birth to evolution.'

Considering the increasingly urgent need for significant change to the education system, there is a strong case to be made that something closer to the Finnish model could be brought about by the introduction of a culture of Compassionate Communities into our schools and colleges. Such a transformation would demand the replacement of prevailing assumptions and expectations with a more humane approach that would require movement in two directions – from the top down and from the ground up – to bring about a co-operative meeting of minds between the education authorities and the teaching staff.

Improved communication and the according of greater recognition for the experience-based evidence that teachers have to offer would bring about a greater degree of confidence and trust. Other necessary changes would then flow from that to improve the morale of both teachers and pupils. Given that greater degree of support, teachers would be strengthened in their self-respect and measures could be devised to alleviate the strains under which they presently work. In such benign circumstances, the overall culture of schools would begin to change in ways that would make them happier, safer and more satisfying environments for all who work and study there. Chances are that academic performance would also improve. But there is still more that could be accomplished.

Whatever else they do, schools help to form – for better or worse – the moral character, values and expectations of the children who attend them. In so doing, they influence the shape of the future. To be truly effective, the introduction of a compassionate culture would significantly improve every aspect of a school's life – what happens in the classroom, in the playground, in the staff room, the dining hall, in the meetings between parents and teachers – and its relations with the surrounding community. It would build on the understanding that the support of family, friends and others is a deeply meaningful factor in a contented human life, and that this is as true for children as it is for adults. For that reason, one of the principal aims of a compassionate culture would be to help pupils to develop and improve the quality of peer relationships and to begin to create their own culture of compassionate relationships in ways that will serve them well in both their present and their future lives.

A current example of how such a pattern of education can be successfully put into practice is evident in the achievements of the Pushkin Trust in Northern Ireland. The trust was founded by Sacha, Duchess of Abercorn, at the time when violence between the deeply divided communities of the province was at its height. Deeply concerned by the traumatic effects of that violence on the lives of children, Sacha devised an educational scheme to bring together pupils from both Protestant and Catholic schools and use creative writing, other art forms and guided experience of the natural world as a means to give voice to their feelings and stimulate their imaginations.

Lindsay Clarke was among the writers invited to act as a mentor to the scheme and he was so impressed by the way it was encouraging the children to tell different and better stories than those that had seen the streets of Ulster run with blood for three hundred years that he went on to work as a consultant of the trust for almost two decades. During that time, he watched children from both communities learn to trust one another by working and playing well together and saw how teachers, teacher-trainers and civil servants developed and extended the programme with growing enthusiasm in both Ulster and Ireland.

What was achieved by the children had a knock-on effect to their parents and their communities and it significantly contributed to the creation of the atmosphere in which the Northern Ireland peace process proved successful.

Commenting on this, Lindsay says:

The founding impulse behind the trust was the compassion that Sacha felt for the suffering of the children affected by the Troubles. She believed that if there was any hope for a better future in that deadlocked time, it must lie with the children. By encouraging them to find their own voice and opening their hearts to a more fulfilling vision of life, space was created in which their world could begin to change for the better.

In a comment on the work of the trust, one of its patrons, Nobel Laureate Seamus Heaney, said that emanating from the Pushkin Trust is, 'A message in praise of creative joy and psychic integrity, of trust in potential and impatience with cliché, a call to everybody to be more ardently and originally themselves.' That assessment was echoed and affirmed by a pupil who took part in one of the trust's events: 'I loved it all, it was breath-taking. I know I can do much more than I ever thought. It was the best five days of my life.' Surely such joy, rather than abject misery, should be the keynote of a child's education into life?

At ground level, many teachers are already teaching compassionate values and putting them into practice in their classrooms. An impressive example of the transformative effects that such efforts can have even in unpropitious circumstances is provided by the work of Bewick Abel Thompson, the son of Julian Abel, who has successfully developed a compassionate education initiative in the primary school where he now teaches.

Having taught for some time at a school in Frome designed for the education of children with special needs, Bewick took a teaching appointment in the very different urban environment of Bristol where he was given responsibility for the most notoriously unruly class in the school. Describing the task that faced him, and explaining why he thought the Compassionate Communities programme might help those children, he said:

The school is in one of the most deprived areas of the country. There is great diversity in ethnicity and religion. None of the parents of the children I teach were born in the UK. Their English is not brilliant and one of the noticeable things is that the children didn't know how to have conversations. It looked like an opportunity to get children to practice that, and begin to understand other people better, which is really useful in the class-room. It feels important in terms of long-lasting education skills for their future because the children don't seem to know how to acknowledge feelings of vulnerability and how to talk about their other emotions.

Because these are basic human skills, Bewick decided that his programme would focus on the children's emotional literacy. He says, 'They don't have the words to describe the emotions they feel. They have a physical response to something that bubbles up inside them. One of the things that a compassionate education gives is a language to start to gain greater self-awareness and, with it, an understanding of how best to respond to other people.'

Bewick began by working out what words are needed to be able to name and articulate emotions in a more self-aware manner and thus to develop a more empathic awareness of what others might be feeling in a given situation. He helped them to see how recognizing a physical feeling, such as your heart beating and your face becoming flushed, you can understand and recognize the feeling of anger. Once a child understands this, they can become aware of how other people feel that emotion too.

Each table at which the children sat was given a talking stick to be held by the person speaking. Thus equipped, the children went on to discuss what kinds of feeling made the classroom a more pleasant environment to be in. From that arose a greater understanding of which emotions are positive in their effect and which are obstructive. Bewick explains:

> *As a result of these discussions, they decided on their own initiative that it would be a good idea to ask each other every morning how they were feeling. To do this, they settled on three questions: How are you feeling now? What has happened in your morning? And, Can you tell me something that you like? This ritual provided them with a way of touching base each morning as the children asked each other about their welfare and learned to care for each other with greater competence.*

Gradually, the atmosphere of the classroom became much calmer. Children who previously had been disruptive became more relaxed. One particular child, whose behaviour in the previous year had been violently disruptive and who had consistently refused to work, responded in a dramatically positive way to this changed regime. When Bewick spoke to his mother, she said it was like having a different child, one who could now go out on school trips and was kind and caring to his little sister. If someone picked on him in the playground he now simply walked away, whereas previously in such situations he had reacted with such violence that he sometimes drew blood from adults.

Other teachers in the school were astonished by what was happening. Unsurprisingly, in a classroom environment that now felt safer and more peaceful, the children's ability to focus on their work and the quality of their academic performance began to show marked improvement. 'They have made massive gains in their reading within six months,' Bewick says. 'This is the skill most closely linked to awareness and being empathetic. They now understand the emotional tones of what is going on around them and, in general, their understanding in all areas has improved.'

The progress the pupils made was not restricted to the classroom. Having acquired new skills of emotional self-awareness there, the children were now ideally placed to take them out into the playground and into the wider community. 'They were becoming agents of change,' Bewick says, 'and the next step was to introduce them to the skills of conflict resolution and to begin to put them into practice. Equipped in this way, children can become playground monitors to whom other children can come for help when conflicts arise.'

Bewick has been deeply heartened by the children's response to his initiatives:

I have so much hope and feel so positive about what this generation can bring. There are conversations happening among them with a greater degree of awareness than anything I recognize from my own experience in primary school. They are more understanding and more accepting. My engagement with them is not reflective of the world portrayed by the media.

Through his work with disadvantaged children from a diversity of ethnic backgrounds in one of the most hard-pressed areas of the country, Bewick has demonstrated how a compassionate school might attend to the academic needs of its pupils while also nourishing their ability to develop successful and mature human relationships. In that respect, it stands in illuminating contrast to the dismal picture painted by the surveys quoted above.

In the TED talk mentioned earlier, Ken Robinson describes how in Death Valley, California, what appeared to be a permanently arid landscape where no plant life could thrive was briefly transformed by a rare rainstorm. The sudden appearance of a colourful carpet of flora was living proof that the landscape was not dead but dormant.

Here was a metaphor for what might be done to bring about a revival in what has become a largely dysfunctional education system. Like many other teachers, Bewick has been working with an actively compassionate imagination to irrigate the arid landscape of the classroom for which he was given responsibility. The result has been a flowering. Patiently working with children from seriously underprivileged backgrounds, he has helped them to become people who are increasingly self-aware, are more responsive and supportive to each other, and who know how to resolve conflicts when they arise. Such stressful situations occur far less frequently in what is now a calmer space. Meanwhile, the children have helped to make of that space a creative environment in which they have such a degree of personal investment that the quality of their work has significantly improved. So too have attendance figures, presumably because coming to school is now a less scary and miserable, more interesting and engaging experience than once it was.

If many more children were allowed access to such sensitive, life-enlarging opportunities to discover and explore the benefits arising from the skilful practice of emotional literacy they might become harbingers of a better, more convivial world than the one they currently inherit. And what is true of pupils in the earlier stages of education holds true for students at the later stages too.

The rising incidence of mental stress and sexually aggressive behaviour in our universities is a matter of increasing concern and there is a serious need for similarly imaginative work to be done there too. In that respect, the restoration of the dignity and importance of the humanities as a vital area of study would be a significant contribution to the development of a more humane and compassionate culture in universities where their reputation has been somewhat demeaned in recent decades and where budget allocations favour the impersonal, but more profitable, realms of science and technology.

COMPASSIONATE ORGANIZATIONS

Compassion has a role to play in all areas of our lives and certainly should not stop at the workplace door. In purely economic terms, it's well known that companies that look after their staff well are able to demonstrate improved performance in comparison with those that do not. But it's not simply a matter of economic considerations. Benevolent companies have higher staff morale, show reduced levels of anxiety and stress and report a marked decrease in the number of working days lost to sickness. They are also successful in recruiting new workers and retaining staff as a mark of their loyalty to the company.

It's no great surprise that people who work in an organization that treats them with care and respect will appreciate such treatment and consequently prove more likely to be happy in their work and to show greater enthusiasm for it, leading to increased productivity. Additionally, the knowledge that they can count on the support of sympathetic management and the kindness of their colleagues can help workers to cope better with testing times, such as illness and the need for care provision in their home life.

Julian Abel recalls a conversation that illustrates the differing impact on two workers of the different cultural environments in which they were employed. The conversation arose while he was helping a hospice to introduce a Compassionate Communities approach to their practice of care.

> *The staff member I was working with described how she had looked after her father who had died in the previous year. She said that the support she received from the hospice was fantastic. People gave her lifts, covered for her when she needed to take her father to hospital, brought in cakes for them and were incredibly sympathetic.*

The kindness, care and concern made a tremendous difference to both her and her father and continued into her bereavement.

Sometime later she spoke about this experience with a social worker who was visiting the hospice. The social worker said that her father had died in the previous year. But when she let her line manager know that her father had been diagnosed with a terminal illness, his response was to say, 'You can have half a day for the funeral,' and the subject was never mentioned again.

The three principal components of the compassionate workplace are: a clearly established company policy; the provision of listening support and the availability of practical help. We will consider each factor in turn.

Developing a compassionate workplace policy

The successful introduction of a Compassionate Communities programme to any organization will require committed effort from two directions. It will certainly need the active co-operation of, and perhaps also the initial motivation from, the staff working at ground level, but from the start it will also need (and may even begin with) the enthusiastic input and support of senior management working from the top down.

Many companies will already have in place policies to support staff who are undergoing troubled times. However, there is often room for improving these policies and for providing clarity about how support can best be given. In looking to make such improvements, discussions about transforming an organization into a Compassionate Community are often most fruitful when they personalize the experience of what it means to undergo hard times. Many people, including chief executives and those in senior management, will have cared for someone suffering from severe illness or will have been bereaved. Shared recognition of the stress of such experiences, along with consideration of what proved helpful at that difficult time, will help executives to a fuller appreciation that more than merely financial benefits will accrue from becoming a compassionate organization.

Company policies that actively support a compassionate culture in the workplace can be a great help to middle managers who may lack the confidence to give people the benefit of the doubt when they complain that they are experiencing personal difficulties. Because such situations can lead to inequities of treatment and a harsh interpretation of company rules, a compassionate policy will provide guidance on the kinds of issues that demand sensitive support. These might include a sympathetic response to problematic domestic situations, such as divorce or caring for someone with serious health problems. The policy will recognize the need for time off work for planning and attending funerals and will appreciate that job performance may not be at the highest level at such times.

If someone is worrying about what is happening at home and afraid that they might get sacked because the need to give a loved one a lift to hospital will make them late for work, anxiety may well make them less efficient. In such circumstances a compassionate policy would allow for the postponement of a performance review. The policy should allow line managers leeway to make their own assessments of the best way to support a troubled member of their staff and to decide how much time an individual might need away from work in order to meet other responsibilities.

Clearly there are limits to what can be done, and equity has to be applied, but appropriate sensitivity of response, which can be enhanced by a short period of training, is a vital element in the culture of a compassionate workplace.

Listening support in the workplace

People looking for support during hard times usually have a good idea about which of their friends is most likely to be sympathetic. Those they turn to are often naturally gifted in the skill of listening without being judgmental or without feeling the need to offer advice. Often enough, tactful listening is all that's required. After all, not everyone wants to be given advice or to be told how to solve their problems, and such offers can even be a hindrance. As a general rule, less than 5 per cent of a company's workforce is needed to fulfil the role of being a good listener. Thus, in an office staffed by a hundred people, there may be just three or four among them who can undertake an informal listening role. A short period of training in communication skills can be helpful to give such people the confidence to do more effectively what they already do well. Simply having access to someone with whom people feel free to talk over their troubles can be a source of relief and support.

Trained listeners can also be proactive in asking people how they are doing, especially if someone is looking unusually tired or stressed. It might also be encouraging to offer a quiet word of sympathy to a person known to be caring for someone at home. Such small unprompted acts of kindness can make a large difference to a person in need of friendly support.

Once arrangements are made to establish identified listeners in the workplace, it will prove both helpful and useful if they meet regularly as a group, perhaps once a month, to discuss the types of problem that they come across. The group can then share knowledge of what has worked well when people came to talk to them, thus pooling their skills and experience in ways which will be mutually supportive.

Practical help in the workplace

Workers have many skills and resources other than those required by their job and developing a bank of the kind of support on offer can be a good way of making them more immediately available for mutual assistance. Thus, an informed listener might post a list of tasks to be covered either in the workplace while someone is away, or domestic chores they need help with at a time of bereavement, for example, whether it be picking up children from school or mowing the lawn. The effect is somewhat similar to the approach discussed in the chapter on creating compassionate networks.

Not everyone feels comfortable in making bold statements of support and most of us are embarrassed if we feel, for whatever reason, unable to respond to a request for help. The existence of a list makes it easier for a person to volunteer the help they feel they can comfortably manage. Such individual acts of kindness can make a big difference when they are added together collectively across the workforce.

Companies working in a neighbourhood that has already developed a training programme for community connectors may find that some members of the workforce already know how to use the local service directory and can direct others to appropriate community support should they need it. People are generally willing to help each other out of a natural sense of compassion, but that is often done more easily when there is access to the informational resources of a service directory. There is no reason why whole workforces cannot become community connectors through a brief training course in the workplace. Simply having useful information at their fingertips makes it much easier for people to offer positive suggestions when listening to a friend or colleague who is going through difficult times.

COMPASSION IN LOCAL GOVERNMENT

Here again, the Somerset town of Frome offers a working model of a viable alternative to long-established conventional practice.

The town boasts a long, sometimes turbulent history of political rebellion, vigorous disputation and non-conformist thought. (Despite the success of his Methodist mission there, John Wesley described it as 'quarrelsome Frome' and a dismayed Anglican curate called it 'a grand hive of schism'.) So it's perhaps not greatly surprising that, in 2011 – a time of increasing disillusionment with established politics and politicians – a group of independently minded Frome people ill-at-ease with the partisan-based structure of a low-energy town council should have decided that the time for change was overdue.

What they had in mind was an attempt to replace a conventional pattern of local government, which was evidently no longer fit for purpose, with a more inclusive democratic process that would be responsive to local needs and experience and would grow from the grassroots up. It would be founded on the belief that human nature tends towards co-operation rather than to confrontation, and it would try to show that democracy will thrive best when faith is placed in the strength and wisdom of the communities it serves.

In his book, *Flatpack Democracy: A Guide to Creating Independent Politics,* Peter Macfadyen, a founding member of that group writes:

The people who formed Independents for Frome (IfF) came together because they cared about their local community and wished to focus solely on bringing benefit to Frome. We developed a Way of Working which is not simply to form another party...but to try and invent a process that would drag local decision-making into the twenty-first century. With IfF we maintain that 'Yes' is a better answer then 'No'; that the possibility of making mistakes should be encouraged; that diversity and different views are positive; and that community leadership is about making bold, local decisions.

In 2012, individuals standing as Independents achieved a majority in the town council elections, which meant that no single political party had overall control.

They set about deploying their imaginative energy and resources to help build and support a lively culture of compassionate community. In the process, they brought a renewed sense of local empowerment to the townspeople and improved their quality of life in a wide variety of ways.

When, in 2013, an Independent council was elected on the Isle of Wight, one commentator predicted that, 'Within a matter of weeks the Independent group will be fighting like rats in a sack and whoever is charged with trying to keep the group together will be at a nervous breakdown point before long.' That did not turn out to be the case in Frome where the contribution of the Independents to the life of the town won such enthusiastic respect that, in the election of 2019, all the seats on the council were won by independent candidates who brought a diversity of perspectives and opinions to the tasks that faced them.

Critical to such success as the IfF council has been able to achieve is its Way of Working. Peter Macfadyen describes this in a list of eight guiding principles designed to further the overall aims of the common cause which is the welfare of Frome. Prefaced by a quotation from the Danish scientist and poet, Piet Hein – 'The noble art of losing face may one day save the human race' – the list requires:

- A willingness and ability to participate in rational debate leading to a conclusion.
- Understanding the difference between constructive debate and personal attacks.
- Avoidance of identifying ourselves so personally with a particular position that this in itself excludes constructive debate.
- Preparedness to being swayed by the argument of others and admitting mistakes.
- Relative freedom from any underlying dogma or ideology which would preclude listening to the views of others.
- Trust, confidence and optimism in other people's expertise and knowledge.
- Confidence in the mechanisms and processes of decision-making that we establish, accepting that the decisions of the majority are paramount.
- An acceptance that 'you win some, you lose some'; it's usually nothing personal and there's really no point in taking defeats to heart.

The council was happy to find that its Way of Working largely corresponded to the Bell Principles of Independent Politics formulated by Martin Bell, who had been elected as an Independent MP on an anti-corruption ticket. That document was designed as a guide to national politics, but its stated principles of integrity, accountability, transparency, honesty and ethical commitment to non-discriminatory pluralism, while listening and 'consulting our communities constantly and innovatively', apply with equal force and urgency to the business of local government.

But those principles are rigorous in their demands, and discussion, negotiation and decision-making remain complex and difficult processes. That is especially the case where there can be no hard-line party discipline and greater public involvement and consultation is encouraged while trying to reach local decisions in response to local interests. For that reason, the Independent councillors of Frome have found it essential and invaluable to engage the help of a neutral facilitator skilled in group work to monitor the proper conduct of their processes.

Reflecting on the council's way of thinking independently together, Sheila Gore, a resident of Frome for 21 years and a town councillor for four years, says, 'The way you work together is really important. It is not trying to win. What you are trying to do is to reach a consensual decision and, if need be, to step back from your passion and go with a collective proposal that works for the whole rather than the individual.'

Until recently, Sheila was the owner of Frome's busy wholefood shop where she would listen to the many issues people regularly spoke about when they came into the shop. In particular, she became engaged in an eventually successful campaign to prevent the opening of a supermarket in the centre of Frome, a town popular largely because of its many small independent shops. She says:

> Shopping is a social activity when it is done on the small scale. The wholefood shop is on a small street without cars going up it, so kids can be left outside, not near a road, and the whole street becomes a much more congenial place to visit. I thought it was important to keep the supermarket out of the town centre in order to retain its character, and I felt the town council were not really listening to the people of Frome.

When elected as a councillor herself, Sheila discovered that she had been mistaken about the council's indifference and became so committed to its work that she eventually agreed to become mayor for a year in order to get better insight into the variety of different groups active in the town. 'The town councillors who become a mayor get to see the town in a different way,' she says. 'I would never have gone to see the Rotary Club or the Lions, who do an amazing amount of integrative work across the town, if I hadn't been mayor. I wouldn't have had access to them.'

Sheila describes the important part played by the town council in stimulating the vitality of Frome's community life:

The council could see the value of the work done by Jenny Hartnoll, who had been developing connections between individual people and groups across Frome for years, and we wanted to support her work, so we funded the trainers for the community connectors. Because we were committed to listening to the community, we ran various panels in the town, and one of them was on health and well-being. Jenny came to the panel meeting along with repre-sentatives from many organizations. The strongest feedback we received was that the many groups already doing a huge number of activities in the community wanted to be connected up. The scheme of establishing community connectors has helped enor-mously in that respect.'

Sheila points out that the council has always been equally conscious of the social impact made by any development to the physical infrastructure of the town.

There is a park run by the town council where we recently put in a beautiful garden area with benches. Mendip Council have a park which is just a grass space with nobody on it. It was not cultivated. We ran a community consultation on what people wanted in the park. Some people wanted an outdoor gym, some wanted play equipment. What people voted for was the planting of an orchard, and so, using our People's Budget [the proportion of the council budget which is spent in accordance with the wishes of the people], that's what we did. It's now an attractive social space used for dog walking where children play. People came up with the ideas and have seen a visible change taking place.

That story exemplifies the way in which the people who live in a community are best placed to determine what's important to them and then devise the best solutions. Open consultation between the people and the council and other statutory bodies is often the best way to get things done. As Sheila says, it's a matter of working with people, not doing something to them.

CHANGING THE WAY THINGS ARE DONE IN CIVIC AFFAIRS

Individuals and organizations are the mainstay of compassionate activity in a society, but their efforts alone are not enough to bring about the widespread cultural changes required for the realization of a comprehensive pattern of compassionate community life. This book has argued that compassionate interaction should be a procreative force at the heart of the way people relate to each other in every aspect of their lives, but for that to happen in a coherent and durably successful manner, there will need to be significant changes in the assumptions and processes by which communities order their public affairs.

Given the rancorous divisions and general air of dysfunctionality that currently prevail like a toxic cloud of pessimism over many areas of human activity, this may sound like a fanciful aspiration, but in a broad range of environments practical steps are already being taken to bring this about.

At the time of writing this book in 2019, a number of cities and towns from across five continents have already committed to making compassion the fundamental value at the civic level. A programme for what this means in practice is provided by the Compassionate City Charter devised by Alan Kellehear. The specific terms of the charter arose out of its author's particular concern with the social issues arising out of serious illness and the need for palliative end-of-life care. By extension, however, its provisions also speak to ways in which a compassionate city would respond to the difficulties caused by the many other testing moments which life can inflict on us.

The charter defines a compassionate city as a community that recognizes that care for one another at times of health crisis and personal challenge is not simply a task solely for health and social services – it is everyone's responsibility. It goes on to state that:

> *Though local government strives to maintain and strengthen quality services for the most fragile and vulnerable in our midst, those persons are not the limits of our experience of fragility and vulnerability. Serious personal crises of physical or mental illness, dying, death and loss may visit any of us, at any time during the normal course of our lives. A compassionate city is a community that squarely recognizes and addresses this social fact.*

For fuller reference, a slightly adapted text of the charter will be found as an appendix to this book (see page 216).

Meanwhile, it's important to note that, within the United Kingdom, Plymouth, Inverclyde and the whole country of Wales have adopted the Compassionate City Charter. Cologne in Germany and a number of cities in Spain have committed to the programme, and cities in Canada, Brazil, Argentina and Colombia have made related initiatives. A well-established programme has been successfully at work in Kerala for more than 12 years.

SPREADING THE WORD

Public engagement is a key component in building a lively culture of Compassionate Communities. Through hearing about and experiencing the benefits of enlarged social relationships, people come to realize how transformative they can be, and it's essential that the message of its personal and social value is shared with the local population. As Jenny Hartnoll's work has demonstrated, imaginative use of media is an effective method of raising public awareness, whether this is through television, radio, social media such as Twitter and Facebook, or local newspapers. Communal spaces, such as museums, galleries and leisure centres also have a role to play in this. As the Compassionate City Charter recommends, the arrangement of annual exhibitions related to themes of compassion can have a powerful effect in changing people's hearts and minds, and thereby enriching the quality of their lives.

FORMATION OF STEERING COMMITTEES

Working from the ground upwards is a foundational principle for the building of Compassionate Communities, but its implementation can be supported from the top down, and the formation of a steering committee to provide support and guidance as the project progresses and develops is a way of securing widespread engagement. Such a committee can be local, regional or national, with members drawn from a wide variety of backgrounds, each bringing their own particular skills and knowledge. Because the presence of a senior public servant in the lead role can help to win widespread support, the Compassionate City Charter recommends that the mayor's office or an equivalent body is a good place to start.

The local chambers of commerce are often made up from senior business leaders in an area and their active involvement can help to persuade local companies to become compassionate organizations. Should a region or nation commit to a culture of Compassionate Communities, then the co-operation of large corporations employing thousands of people would set a good example and encourage other business to follow suit.

Compassion is a value endorsed by many religions, so it would also be helpful to have representation from religious organizations on a steering committee. All over the world, religious communities are proactively running initiatives to help vulnerable people. While caring for their own believers should be a matter of routine, the provision of care for non-believers without expectation of return can be a still great propagator of compassion. Through simple word of mouth, the religious communities in a neighbourhood can help to identify and aid those who are sick or in need, along with the frail and elderly whose lack of social mobility may mean that their situations otherwise pass unnoticed. Many people use religious leaders for funeral services, and if a church or temple were to set up a bereavement group, people suffering from recent loss could meet and socialize and make others aware of the existence of such invaluable support.

As Sheila Gore's mayoral activities in Frome demonstrate, politicians usually have access to strong connections in community life, and because they can be a persuasive voice in winning wider engagement they too should be part of a steering committee. At the very least, politicians should be known for their kindness, and an unwillingness to promote this most basic of human values would indicate that they are not fit to serve the people who voted for them.

Councils are key bodies in deciding how the resources accruing from government funding and local taxation will be invested, so they too need to be represented on the steering committee. Because they tend to focus mainly on physical infrastructure as a means to stimulate local economies, they often overlook urgent needs for investment in social infrastructure, despite it being an important part of their responsibility.

Planning applications, for example, can have a profound effect on the quality of social relationships. As Sheila's experience in Frome indicates, supermarkets have become expert in persuading local planning committees to allow them to build large stores on the outskirts of towns. The consequence has been the depletion of town centres which too often have little more to offer than banks, estate agencies and thrift shops. The loss of a wider range of shops not only marks the death of many small businesses, it also reduces opportunities for social exchange while people are out shopping.

If not carefully managed with an eye to the greater good, the planning of road networks can also have undesirable effects. In his TED talk, Mick Cornett tells of, 'How an Obese Town Lost a Million Pounds'. When he was elected mayor of Oklahoma City in the United States, it had the unenviable reputation of housing the highest levels of obesity in the country. He realized that while the city had built good facilities for the populace, no walkways had been built to connect them. Furthermore, the road network made it difficult even to cross the road. Simply by shifting the focus of investment in infrastructure and thus making the city an easier place for people to navigate on foot, the inhabitants managed collectively to lose one million pounds in weight between 2004 and 2012. An effective steering commitment for the development of a Compassionate Community would draw attention to such issues and their possible consequences whenever any plans for infrastructure, both physical and social, were being made.

Because educational institutions that adopt a compassionate approach can have an influential role to play in developing a livelier sense of compassionate community, leading educators would be valuable members of a steering committee. Media representation would also be needed to promote greater awareness of the very concept of Compassionate Communities as a feasible and desirable possibility and then to publicize the benefits of its effects.

As things stand, media organizations tend to focus on negative or disastrous aspects of the world's news. 'If it bleeds, it leads' has long been a catchphrase among editors, but such a disproportionately alarming selection of stories from each day's events creates a picture of the world as far more dangerous than it actually is and thus aggravates the general epidemic of anxiety and fear. Lamentably, this distorted image of the world is often used by politicians to manipulate populations for their own ends. Were media leaders from radio, television and newspapers to participate in the deliberations of a steering committee working towards the adoption of Compassionate Communities programmes, they might have a better understanding of the need to give regular coverage to the positive impacts of what can be achieved by the compassionate aspect of the human imagination.

This is by no means an exhaustive list of the kind of people who could usefully serve on a steering committee, and selection always depends on local preferences, needs and concerns. It is important however not to wait for everyone to be on board before making a start. To do so might mean that the initiative is aborted, either through bureaucratic delay or because a new, less sympathetic bunch of politicians has taken over, in which case the process of winning the necessary support would have to begin all over again. That might take years. Better to gather together a core group of people who are strongly motivated to get an initiative going and then invite others to join as the momentum of the project gradually builds.

Meanwhile, more ambitiously, at a national level, whole governments might commit to the active adoption of compassionate programmes of action. The national government itself could, and should, become a compassionate employer, and it should routinely use the value of compassion as a standard to assess the likely impact of its policy decisions on people's lives.

In our currently volatile and divisive political circumstances that might sound fanciful, but there is an encouraging example of such progress already in action: at the time of writing, the Compassionate City Charter is being adapted for use by the government of Wales and is currently passing through all the major departments for approval.

CHAPTER 10

THE POLITICS OF COMPASSION

We often think of peace as the absence of war, that if powerful countries would reduce their weapon arsenals, we could have peace. But if we look deeply into the weapons, we see our own minds – our own prejudices, fears and ignorance. Even if we transport all the bombs to the moon, the roots of war and the roots of bombs are still there, in our hearts and minds, and sooner or later we will make new bombs. To work for peace is to uproot war from ourselves and from the hearts of men and women.

Thich Nhat Hanh, *Living Buddha, Living Christ*

In 2019, a report put together for the United Nations by 450 experts from 50 countries warned that more than a million species of plants and animals are under threat of extinction, that more than half a million species on land 'have insufficient habitat for long-term survival', that the oceans are in a similarly critical condition and that human behaviour is responsible for this imminently catastrophic damage. The report urges world leaders to take immediate action to halt the decline because there is still time to save the environment on which our own survival also depends. That will only be done if governments, companies and individuals change their behaviour in ways that prioritize the urgent need to protect the planet's biodiversity and eco-systems.

Meanwhile, the gravity of the situation is made still more alarming by the lack of significant action being taken to limit carbon emissions and thereby reduce the disastrous environmental effects of global warming. Cynically manipulated political systems serve the interests of the already powerful and wealthy and the currently dominant economic policies of the world seem purpose-built to widen the already outrageous size of the gap between the extremely rich and the increasingly poor. Against such grim and seemingly unstoppable trends, the power of human compassion may seem too frail an instrument to bring about the necessary processes of change. But the global case for compassion is not without hope.

When, in a letter to Thomas Mercer, the philosopher Edmund Burke said that, 'All it takes for evil to flourish is for good men to do nothing,' he was implicitly asserting that the actions of individuals *can* have positive results. Time and again, history has certainly shown that their failure to act can prove disastrous, so this chapter will consider ways in which the actions of individuals can bring about social change and influence those who are most resistant to change. That latter challenge presents peculiar difficulties because, as the American writer Upton Sinclair pointed out, 'It is difficult to get a man to understand something when his salary depends upon his not understanding it.'

Concentration on the acquisition of wealth, however, is unlikely to successfully address the grave issues outlined above. Nor is it even a guarantor of individual happiness. A shift of national focus away from persistent ambitions of economic growth and the statistics of gross domestic product will offer a much better chance of improving – both for individuals and for the planet as a whole – the overall quality of life and even, ultimately, the likelihood of our survival.

But how, in a world addicted to the acquisition of material goods (and even of money for its own sake) might such a shift be made? Is it even possible?

The small Himalayan kingdom of Bhutan may already have pointed the way.

In place of an obsessive preoccupation with GDP, that country has developed a scale of 'gross national happiness' as a means to assess the well-being and contentment of the population. The criteria by which that is measured are: psychological well-being, health, time use, education, cultural diversity and resilience, good governance, community vitality and ecological diversity and resilience, along with general standards of living.

In stark contrast with those humane points of reference, the OECD (Organization for Economic Co-operation and Development) definition of gross domestic product, which is used as a proxy marker for well-being and happiness by many nations, is: 'an aggregate measure of production equal to the sum of the gross values added of all resident and institutional units engaged in production and services (plus any taxes), and minus any subsidies, on products not included in the value of their outputs'. The nature of the abstract, depersonalized language employed by that definition is itself a marker of the essential difference between the two scores.

The contrast between these two visions of the world not only begs the fundamental question of what values most deeply matter to us, it also requires us to consider in practical terms which of the two is likeliest to generate a sense of happiness and contentment in human communities and create the kind of circumstances in which the natural order can thrive.

The shift to a more rounded view of the deep sources of general happiness and welfare is as important on an individual level as it is to enhancing the chances of achieving world peace and ensuring those of planetary survival. The challenge is how to turn a personal commitment to compassionate motivation and action into a political force that will change the course of destructive human behaviour.

COMPASSION AND SELF-INTEREST

As human beings, we need to feel we belong to social groups that give support, meaning and value to our existence. That need has shaped our biochemistry, our behaviour and our patterns of culture and survival – patterns into which children are educated and which are passed on, in evolving form, from generation to generation. But all social groups need measures of order and control to hold them together, and throughout history ruling elites have emerged to maintain that order, usually to enforce it to their own advantage.

There is a direct correlation between the degree of compassion that an individual is capable of showing to others and the countervailing degree of that person's active self-centredness. Social dominance orientation is a score used to quantify this correlation, with people who have high scores tending to be more predisposed to violence, racism, prejudice and a lack of compassion. Unsurprisingly, those people who feel the strongest craving for the accumulation of personal wealth and power for its own sake, and who are resolute to act on that craving, will tend to be among the least compassionate. In pursuit of their ambitions, such people often find themselves faced by the temptation – or what they might perceive as the acceptable necessity – to compromise their moral conduct, forgo their personal integrity, and sacrifice the interests of others and those of what might generally be considered the greater good.

At the root of the conflict between the claims of compassion and those of self-interest is a fundamental question of the values by which we choose to live. Such conflicts are, of course, played out daily in the lives of many individuals, but they are likely to prove more intense, and have more far-reaching consequences, in the lives of people occupying positions of authority. Their opportunities for obtaining access to power and wealth are greater than for most of us, while their privileged circumstances make it easier to manipulate the often complex processes by which such material advantages can be achieved.

Whatever their nature, and whether their advantage is based in religion, politics, class or caste, such elites have historically deployed similar strategies to justify their position and authority. They are the guardians of the myths and rituals that give shape and coherence to a society and thus constitute the sense of reality within which its people live. The myth might be that of the divine right to rule, that of government of the people, by the people, for the people, or whatever other pattern of belief or ideology secures the assent and allegiance of the majority of the population. But, as the old saying has it, power corrupts and absolute power corrupts absolutely, so, regrettably and perhaps inevitably, the stratagems employed by elites to hold on to their power – dynastic succession, nepotism, patronage, persecution, suppression, secrecy and censorship among them – tend towards corruption. In its most corrosive forms, such corruption puts personal interests, or those of a ruling group, above the greater good of humanity. Which is to say that its actions are, at heart, deficient in compassion.

When people in positions of authority act in a manner that causes harm to others, they have disregarded compassion as a motivating value that should stand high on the list of considerations that need to be taken into account whenever decisions are made in politics, business, health affairs, education or any other matter that has a significant impact on the general quality of life.

Nor does this ethical standard apply only in so far as it affects the human realm. The UN report on the perilous condition of the planet's biodiversity and ecosystems is not just an admonition that we should behave more responsibly in the interests of our own survival, it is a devastating confession of a worldwide human failure of compassion in relation to the other species with which we share this planet's gift of life. Equipped with larger brain power and formidable technological force, we have set ourselves up as the powerful ruling elite and allowed our ambitions and appetites, along with our baser emotions of greed and fear, to determine the fate of countless species and condemn them to death.

Whether recognized or not by the courts, ecocide is an existential crime, characterized as much by a catastrophic failure of compassion as were the many atrocious acts of genocide witnessed during the past century. It is as much a sign of moral corruption, and without serious and urgent action to put right this planetary scale of wrongs, efforts to act in all the other areas to which this book draws attention will eventually prove to have been in vain. But here, as elsewhere, a renewed and deeper evaluation of compassion as the essential driving force is the corrective antidote. Its application, both in personal resolve and larger group action, can help us to overcome those darker emotions that permit us to act in ways that turn out, in the long run, to be self-destructive.

POLITICAL STRUCTURES AND THE FOUR PILLARS OF ELITISM

Those who have most to lose are likeliest to resist change, and in his book *The Prostitute State: How Britain's Democracy Has Been Bought*, Donnachadh McCarthy describes how four pillars of elitism work together to maintain the benefits which they feel they earn and deserve.

The first pillar is that of corrupted democracy in which the interests and activities of corporate lobbyists and politicians have become deeply intertwined. The alliance is sealed by the corporate funding of political parties and by a convenient arrangement of revolving doors that allows ease of job movement between politics and industry.

The second pillar is that of a prostituted academia, in which those vested interests seek to determine both the agendas of an education system that they partially fund and the character of the research it conducts. This process has become intertwined with those of corrupted democracy, and much academic research has become so compromised that papers advancing a particular view are routinely funded by corporate organizations in their efforts to maximize their profits.

The third pillar is that of criminal tax havens where money from across the world is deposited by corrupt individuals and businesses with little in the way of effective international protest and opposition. Trillions of dollars are stolen and hoarded by already wealthy businessmen and politicians prepared to rob the state they represent without any apparent concern for the ways in which that money might benefit millions of people who have barely enough food and water to survive. As a consequence of such indifference, grotesque differentials in prosperity prevail worldwide. In the USA in 2017, 1 per cent of the population had more money than the remaining 99 per cent, while globally, 38 per cent of the world's entire wealth was owned by 1 per cent of the people.

The fourth and final pillar is that of the prostituted media. In the UK, five billionaires currently own 80 per cent of all media outlets. To quote McCarthy's summary of this lamentable state of affairs, 'If the rich elites and corporations control the production of thought, the dissemination of thought, the implementation of thought and the funding of thought, then we no longer live in a democracy but in The Prostitute State.'

JOINING FORCES FOR COMPASSIONATE CHANGE

A sober consideration of such compromised circumstances, along with an awareness of the frequently disastrous course of history and the potentially catastrophic environmental crisis across the globe, can generate disabling feelings of impotence and hopelessness. But, as was said earlier, we are the case for hope as well as the authors of our own despair, and if our prospects for the future are to be improved, it will be as the result of transformational action taken by responsible individuals and the committed groups that they combine to form. For those efforts to succeed, our rational faculties will need to work in fruitful co-operation with our capacity for fellow feeling, and in building such a comprehensive alliance of heart, head and hand, the strength of the compassionate imagination will provide a powerful engine of change.

Fortunately, we have two great current examples of active hope which provide valuable lessons on how change across whole systems can come about. The first is provided by professor of political science Gene Sharp's account in his book *From Dictatorship to Democracy* of how his non-violent methods were used to overthrow oppressive dictatorships. The second is that of Greta Thunberg and the environmental group Extinction Rebellion, which has recruited growing numbers of people worldwide to take direct action demanding that governments make a serious and urgent commitment to address the accelerating environmental crisis. In the process they are making use of some of the methods of non-violent civil disobedience recommended by Gene Sharp.

In his book Gene Sharp shows that the continuing existence of a totalitarian regime depends on its compliant acceptance by the people it subjugates. His analysis of the process by which governments command such assent identifies the following key factors:

- The establishment of belief in its legitimacy as a moral authority to be obeyed
- The number and importance of those willing to co-operate with its rule
- The command of the requisite skills and knowledge
- The employment of psychological and ideological methods
- The control of the necessary material resources
- The employment of punitive sanctions against resistance

All of these factors are dependent on the passive assent of the subjugated population, but that assent can be withdrawn. As Machiavelli long ago warned, a prince 'who has the public as a whole for his enemy can never make himself secure; and the greater his cruelty, the weaker does his regime become.'

In his extraordinary book, which is freely available online, Sharp lists two hundred essentially non-violent strategies of civil disobedience which have been used to overthrow totalitarian regimes. These methods have been successfully employed in widely different circumstances, sometimes causing regimes to collapse in a matter of weeks. The fall of the Berlin Wall in East Germany, the popular revolution in Romania and the events of the Arab Spring furnish notable examples.

However, it's important to be aware that the dynamics by which totalitarian regimes dominate their people are also subtly at play in existing democracies.

They are clearly active in the way that business corporations control the economic and, to some degree, the cultural life of nations, as is demonstrated by McCarthy's analysis of the four pillars of the Prostitute State. Yet, by the same token, the strategies that have overthrown totalitarian regimes can be effectively put to work in this context too.

The creation of a nationwide sense of Compassionate Community will demand a radical change in the currently prevailing system of values. Charismatic thinkers and courageous leaders will emerge to articulate that need for change, yet however eloquent the power of disparate and un-coordinated voices (even those of world-famous celebrities), their influence can swiftly dissipate. If we are to find our way through the mire of bitter division, anger, resentment, discontent, hatred, violence, depression and suffering that presently characterizes the daily news of the world towards a more convivial and ultimately more meaningful way of life, then imaginative, non-violent action must be taken by increasing numbers of people for whom compassion has become a fundamental value in their lives.

As Greenpeace, Amnesty International and aid organizations such as the Red Cross have demonstrated, each in their different ways, prolonged campaigns with developed communication strategies are more likely to be successful. But for humane values to become an effective political force for change, strategic programmes of action, such as those employed by Extinction Rebellion, must be organized and implemented. In that way, where violent revolutions have failed or merely created more problems than they solved, a non-violent, population-based, ground-up movement of compassion could further a desperately needed evolution of consciousness and bring about a benevolent process of social change.

THE POLITICS OF COMPASSION

Cynical self-interest is a corrosive feature in politics across the world and, as a consequence, the general public has itself become more cynical about politicians and the way that government business is conducted. Governments have rarely been transparent about their activities but we live in times when investigative journalism makes it difficult to keep things permanently under cover and, for most people, the exposure of political corruption in public affairs, whether driven by personal or party interests, is deeply shocking.

Such figures would do well to contemplate the cautionary words about the abuse of power and the consequences of warfare uttered by the ancient Chinese philosopher, Chuang Tzu (translated by Thomas Merton):

> *...Should you seem to succeed,*
> *Success itself will bring more conflict.*
> *Why all these guards*
> *Standing at attention*
> *At the palace gate, around the temple altar,*
> *Everywhere?*
>
> *You are at war with yourself!*
> *You do not believe in justice,*
> *Only in power and success.*
> *If you overcome*

An enemy and annex his country
You will be even less at peace
With yourself than you are now.
Nor will your passions let you
Sit still. You will fight again
And again for the sake of
A more perfect exercise of 'justice'!

In contrast, the deeply moving speech given by Prime Minister Jacinda Ardern in response to the March 2019 bombings in Christchurch, New Zealand, insists that a politics of compassion is both feasible and essential. Speaking at the National Memorial Service, she said:

What words adequately express the pain and suffering of 50 men, women and children lost, and so many injured? I thought there were none. And then I came here and was met with this simple greeting. As-salaam Alaikum. Peace be upon you. They were words spoken by a community who, in the face of hate and violence, had every right to express anger but instead opened their doors for all of us to grieve with them. And so we say to those who have lost the most, we may not have always had the words. We may have left flowers, performed the haka, sung songs or simply embraced. But even when we had no words, we still heard yours, and they have left us humbled and they have left us united.

Over the past two weeks we have heard the stories of those impacted by this terrorist attack. They were stories of bravery. They were stories of those who were born here, grew up here, or who had made New Zealand their home who had sought refuge, or sought a better life for themselves or their families. These stories now form part of our collective memories. They will remain with us forever. They are us. But with that memory comes a responsibility. A responsibility to be the place that we wish to be. A place that is diverse, that is welcoming, that is kind and compassionate. Those values represent the very best of us…

Our challenge now is to make the very best of us, a daily reality. Because we are not immune to the viruses of hate, of fear of other. We never have been. But we can be the nation that discovers the cure. And so to each of us as we go from here, we have work to do, but do not leave the job of combatting hate to the government alone. We each hold the power, in our words and in our actions, in our daily acts of kindness. Let that be the legacy of 15 March. To be the nation we believe ourselves to be…

The world has been stuck in a vicious cycle of extremism breeding extremism and it must end. We cannot confront these issues alone, none of us can. But the answer to them lies in a simple concept that is not bound by domestic borders, that isn't based on ethnicity, power base or even forms of governance. The answer lies in our humanity.

Those words were occasioned by extraordinary events of appalling cruelty, but they apply with equal force to the way in which we conduct ourselves in our daily lives. They are both a testament to, and an urgent plea for, an active politics of compassion.

IN CONCLUSION

The alarming proliferation of the coronavirus from continent to continent has increased consciousness of the already daunting planetary scale of the problems which now face us as a species. Many of those problems are, of course, self-created and they have now reached calamitous proportions. But whether confronting the ravages of the Covid-19 disease or acknowledging the damage done to the environment which sustains our life by our violation of natural laws, the true disaster now would be for men and women of good will to throw up their hands in despair and become complicit with the self-defeating conspiracy of cynicism, hypocrisy and wilful ignorance that darkens so much of the cultural landscape today.

Paradoxically, the coronavirus, which presents such a threat to our way of life, seems in many ways to be good for the health of the planet. The enforced closing of industrial plants and the reduction of aviation and motorised traffic have markedly reduced carbon emissions. The air in cities is more breathable and there are even reports that fish have returned to the suddenly clearer waters of the Venice canals.

These desirable changes have come about because fast-tracked research has shown how the coronavirus thrives on close personal contact, and that its progress can be slowed only by public efforts to reduce such contact. But the success of governmental measures relies on a general willingness to accept the strict limitations they impose on individual freedom. In these stressful circumstances the chilly term 'social distancing' has quickly entered common speech.

The difficulty arises from the fact that human beings are essentially social animals, and there are good reasons for this beyond the simple pleasure we take in keeping company. This book has drawn attention to medical research which shows that good social relationships are fundamental to our health and welfare. They offer better treatment for hypertension than medication, and are more effective at reducing the risk of death than losing weight, improving diet, and stopping smoking or drinking. Such research is the product of collaborative activity, which is the way human beings learn from each other. That we can do so even with limited face-to-face communication is a huge advantage – not least because it's emotionally important to us that we find ways to stay in touch when we are kept apart. This means that even as we dutifully practice social distancing, we also need to come closer together. To do that will be much easier if we create, and live within, an active sense of compassionate community.

There are obvious practical reasons for that, such as the provision of support for isolated individuals in need of food, warmth and care. But, as this book has tried to show, it's also the case that through compassionate behaviour people improve their own health and well-being, particularly the strength of their immune system. Whether consciously or not, an intuitive understanding of that fact lies behind the many successful efforts through which, in this time of crisis, both individuals and communities have fostered good relationships while respecting the restrictions imposed by the pandemic.

Examples of this are widespread. At the simplest level, people do it by chatting with neighbours (perhaps for the first time) over the garden fence or when separated by a window. Inspired by the beleaguered Italians who lifted their spirits by singing together from their balconies, 'sofa choirs' began to sing together over the internet – one of the many ways in which modern technology has come to our aid. Even members of the older generation not fluent with the use of laptops and smartphones have been taught by a compassionate network of family or friends to connect virtually to their usual social groups and perhaps to find new ones.

Compassion is a life-enhancing act of imagination and crisis generates inventive activity. Across the world, individuals and communities have responded creatively to the challenges posed by this pandemic with that spontaneous warmth of heart. Such responses are particularly important when the Covid-19 infection ends in death. Even in normal times bereavement can be a severely depleting condition. When the old and vulnerable are at risk of dying alone, grief may be aggravated by the demands of hygiene and the need for social isolation. After this crisis has passed we may need to observe a national Day of Mourning to alleviate such feelings.

In the meantime, it's important that people stay as emotionally close to one another as physical separation allows. That way we will emerge from this ordeal with a strengthened sense of our common humankindness and with an active understanding that compassion is not only a profound human need, it's the surest foundation for a sane, healthy and decent community life.

Taking as its starting point the very real changes that were made in Frome a number of years before the present planetary crisis began, this book has sought to make a strong case for hope founded on the innate human capacity for compassion. Beyond all divisions of gender, nationality, race, political opinion, religious belief and cultural practices, that capacity is a universal bond between us all. It is on the deep ground of that commonality that our survival as a species will ultimately depend.

We know that our present way of life is both inequitable and unsustainable. We know that change is inevitable, either in the form of some collective human or ecological disaster and ensuing worldwide conflict, or – more positively – as a result of an urgently needed evolutionary shift in human consciousness and behaviour.

As we have tried to show, the adoption of compassion as a ruling principle calls into question many aspects of the way in which we currently live, and on which an abiding, if illusory, sense of our security has been founded. It will, therefore, meet with resistance, and that will only be overcome by the joint persuasive action of many people working together for the common good. But such action begins with the choices that individual people make, so the responsibility for change primarily rests with each of us.

Catastrophes of our own making come about when we choose to ignore the fact that what our human hopes and needs have in common far outweighs our differences. We all inhabit a body with its strengths and mortal frailties; we are all eventually prey to illness and death; and sooner or later we are all faced either with the need for the compassionate attention that others can give, or the need to afford such care to those we love. But when individuals begin to pool their skills and resources in imaginative ways, and act courageously together, the scale of their success is vastly increased.

A culture which privileges compassion as its prevailing value will allow individuals to flourish and freely bring their personal talents and gifts to the communities in which they live. Unanticipated possibilities will then emerge, presenting new ways of addressing what may previously have appeared to be insoluble problems. In such benevolent circumstances, hearts are lifted and the case for hope is more strongly made. And as the people who work together in this way begin to change the world immediately around them, so too, however gradually, the wider world beyond begins to change.

A MANIFESTO FOR
COMPASSIONATE COMMUNITIES

This manifesto is a call to all people. Recognizing compassion as a fundamental human quality present in all of us, either as a potential or in various stages of realization, this manifesto is a call for the creation of more Compassionate Communities.

We all care for our friends and family. We freely offer kindness and help to both neighbours and strangers in times of trouble, and such care is the basis for friendship and trust. Without this generosity of heart any degree of humane society would simply not be possible. Yet increasingly, across the world, we see societies dominated by greed, envy, intolerance, violence, repression and fear. Such developments reflect a failure of compassion and emotional literacy, both at the individual level and in organized group and state activity.

While calling on individuals to challenge and reject all use of violence and aggression, both personal and public, this manifesto for Compassionate Communities insists on the need for a social movement embodying forms of political activity, which encourage the fundamental values of human compassion in all significant aspects of our lives – in education, business, health and welfare provision, in religion and in politics at local, national and international levels, and in proper care for the natural environment which sustains all our lives.

COMPASSIONATE COMMUNITIES IN THE LIVES OF INDIVIDUALS

Care for one another is the only sane basis of human society. Kindness to our family and friends, our neighbours and our community members is the true basis for quality of life. Individuals have a responsibility to the people around them, and Compassionate Communities call on us all to respect this responsibility. It insists that difficulties must be resolved by a commitment to dialogue and co-operation underpinned by humankindness.

Emotions and desires, whether physical, sexual or psychological, exist as a human reality, but acts of violence and aggression are a failure of compassion and of emotional literacy – a quality that needs to be nurtured from birth to death in all of us. Emotional literacy is a way of respecting the often difficult range of human emotions while not being at their mercy and is a fundamental element in the life of Compassionate Community. It is about caring for others while finding ways to express emotions without causing them physical, sexual or psychological harm. Compassionate Community rejects racism, sexism and other forms of repression at an individual level, while celebrating diversity of race, gender, sexuality, politics and religion in wider society.

COMPASSIONATE COMMUNITIES IN EDUCATION

True education goes beyond the acquisition of knowledge. It has moral and ethical purpose and, for that reason, the development of compassion needs to be included in all educational programmes. This requires education in the values of emotional literacy as the mature way of dealing with difficult emotions while avoiding the harm that they might otherwise cause.

Information is now available to all who have access to electronic media, so the capacity to recall large amounts of remembered knowledge is no longer needed to form harmonious societies. What we need to learn is skill in accessing this information and the understanding of how to use it wisely. Compassion is an act of the sympathetic imagination, so the creative use of the imagination is an ethical skill for our children to acquire if they are to show proper care for others, for their communities and eventually for their own children, while developing informed sensitivity to the natural environment that supports their lives.

COMPASSIONATE COMMUNITIES IN BUSINESSES AND MEDIA

Profit is a prerequisite for businesses to thrive. However, the responsibility of compassionate businesses is not solely to generate profit. Compassionate businesses need to care for their employees. They need to ensure that their activities leave the world in a better state for our children and our children's children. This means ensuring that business methods do not damage the health and welfare of people and the natural environment. Compassionate Communities call on all businesses to adopt and promote compassionate activities, including:

- Compassionate workplace policies which ensure proper care for the welfare and morale of employees, including support at times of stress, ill health and loss
- Environmental care to ensure that business activities support improvement of the environment and act responsibly to avoid or repair any environmental harm
- Rejection of corruption. Corruption is persuasion used in the absence of compassion, regardless of its impact on others. It is a manifestation of greed both in the person giving the

bribe and the person receiving it. It is a failure of compassion and emotional literacy

- By definition, products, such as those of the arms industry, that cause harm to humans and the environment can have no place in the world of Compassionate Communities
- Compassionate Communities call on all forms of media to promote human values of equity, compassion and care, and to desist from the propagation of exploitation, racism and oppression

While recognizing that accumulation of wealth and power is part of human society, Compassionate Communities call on all who have accumulated those advantages to use their assets and resources for the present and future benefit of both the human and natural world around them.

COMPASSIONATE COMMUNITIES IN RELIGION

Spiritual expression is a part of human cultural evolution. Compassionate Communities call on all religions to respect diversity of belief and to embrace compassion and kindness as fundamental human values that transcend differences of creed and practice. Without those values, religion is of no true help either to individuals or societies. Compassionate Communities call for all religions to reject violence of any kind and to cease coercing others to adopt and acquiesce in their beliefs. In place of such aggressive practice, it insists on tolerance and respect for diversity as fundamental moral and spiritual values.

COMPASSIONATE COMMUNITIES IN POLITICS

Politics conducted without compassion causes harm. Compassionate Communities call on all political activity, from individual to national and international state levels, to reject all forms of violence and oppression. It calls on individuals to challenge governments to adopt compassionate policies and promote legislation that improves welfare for all, irrespective of race, cultural diversity, religious belief or gender. National boundaries need to be respected, but not as an end in themselves and should be as open as possible.

A compassionate nation prioritizes the quality of the life of its citizens above the acquisition by the state of influence, power or wealth.

Compassionate politics will:

- Reject violence and oppression of any sort
- Care for the rights and welfare of individuals
- Reject corruption and greed as acceptable means and motive for action
- Because productivity, growth and profit alone are not sufficient value to ensure general welfare, compassionate government will legislate to enable and advance the creation of Compassionate Communities in neighbourhoods, workplaces and educational institutions
- It will embrace renewable resources as the primary means of energy production
- It will care for the environment and the wider well-being of future generations

COMPASSIONATE COMMUNITIES IN HEALTH AND WELFARE

Healthcare is provided solely to benefit humans and not for profit. The pharmaceutical industry has a responsibility to ensure their products do not cause harm and are not sold for the sake of profit alone. Health is not solely about physical well-being. It is also about the need to live securely within a compassionate society.

Compassionate Communities recognize that care for one another at times of health crisis and personal loss is not a task solely for health and social services: it is everyone's responsibility. However, receiving support through testing times also comes with responsibility. Whether rich or poor, individuals in Compassionate Communities commit to improving the quality of life for those around them and to ensuring proper care for the environment in which they live.

COMPASSIONATE COMMUNITIES AND THE ENVIRONMENT

Environmental degradation is our single biggest threat. As is now well established, the danger rises from the use of fossil fuels or other sources of energy that cause environmental damage and from the excessive exploitation of natural resources. Compassionate Communities are committed to the use of renewable energy as a primary source of all energy production. The avoidance of pollution and other forms of damage causing harm to ecological diversity is the responsibility of all individuals, businesses and states. That responsibility includes active concern for the welfare of animals – they too experience emotions and seek happiness. As humans, we have the responsibility to live harmoniously with the life of our planet and its species, making sure that we hand it on to our children in a better state than we found it.

www.resurgence.org

THE COMPASSIONATE CITY CHARTER

The approaches to bringing compassion into civic life are encapsulated in the Compassionate City Charter. The current version is adapted from the charter developed by Professor Allan Kellehear, which is more focused on end-of-life care. The charter outlines a structured approach across 13 domains of civic life that helps to provide focus for those actively concerned in developing community life across a geographical area, whether it be a town, a village, a city or a rural location.

COMPASSIONATE CITIES

Compassionate Cities are communities that publicly recognize and seek to aid these troubled populations by enlisting all the major sectors of a community to help support them and reduce the negative social, psychological and medical impact of serious illness, caregiving and bereavement. It recognizes that it is the responsibility of us all to do so.

Though local government strives to maintain and strengthen quality services for the most fragile and vulnerable in our midst,

215

those persons are not the limits of our experience of fragility and vulnerability. Serious personal crises of physical or mental illness, dying, death and loss may visit any of us, at any time during the normal course of our lives. A Compassionate City is a community that squarely recognizes and addresses this social fact.

Accordingly, the Compassionate Cities Charter makes the following statements and demands:

- Through auspices of the Mayor's office a Compassionate City will – by public marketing and advertising, by use of the city's network and influences, by dint of collaboration and co-operation, in partnership with social media and its own offices – develop and support the following 13 social changes to the city's key institutions and activities.

- Our schools will have annually reviewed policies and guidance documents to develop a compassionate school

- Our workplaces will have annually reviewed policies and guidance documents to develop a compassionate organization

- Our trade unions will have annually reviewed policies and guidance documents to provide compassionate support to members undergoing serious personal crises of physical or mental illness, dying, death and loss

- Our churches and temples will have at least one dedicated group to supporting Compassionate Communities

- Our city's health and social care institutions, including hospitals, hospices and care homes, will have a community development programme, which involves citizens in supporting residents of those institutions

- Our city's major museums and art galleries will hold annual exhibitions on the experiences of crises of physical or mental illness, dying, death and loss and caregiving

- Our city will host an annual memorial parade representing the major sectors of society, to celebrate Compassionate Communities, supporting people undergoing crises of physical or mental illness, dying, death and loss and caregiving

- Our city will create an incentives scheme to celebrate and highlight the most creative compassionate organization, event and individual/s. The scheme will take the form of an annual award administered by a committee. A 'Mayor's Prize' will recognize individual/s for that year, those who most exemplify the city's values of compassionate care

- Our city will publicly showcase, in print and in social media, our local government policies, services, funding opportunities, partnerships, and public events that address 'our compassionate concerns' with living with illness, ageing, life-threatening and life-limiting illness, loss and bereavement, and long-term caring

- Our city will work with local social or print media to encourage an annual city-wide short story or art competition that helps raise awareness of crises of physical or mental illness, dying, death and loss and caregiving

- All our compassionate policies and services, and in the policies and practices of our official compassionate partners and alliances, will demonstrate an understanding of how diversity shapes the experience of ageing, physical or mental illness, dying, death and loss and caregiving – through ethnic, religious, gendered, and sexual identity and through the social experiences of poverty, inequality, and disenfranchisement

- We will seek to encourage and to invite evidence that institutions for the homeless and the imprisoned have support plans in place for crises of physical or mental illness, dying, death and loss and caregiving

- Our city will establish and review these targets and goals in the first two years and thereafter will add one more sector annually to our action plans for a compassionate city – e.g. hospitals, further and higher education, charities, community and voluntary organizations, emergency services, and so on

- This charter represents a commitment by the city to embrace a view of health and wellbeing that embraces community empathy, directly supporting its inhabitants to address the negative health impacts of social inequality and marginalization attributable to physical or mental illness, dying, death and loss and caregiving

The words of the charter remind us that a city is not merely a place to work and shop and access necessary services: it should also be a social environment where, in schools and workplaces, in places of worship and recreation, in cultural forums and social networks anywhere within the city's influence, we can enjoy the pleasure, safety and protection of each other's company. It should be that, for both children and adults, throughout the length of our lives.

www.compassionate-communities.co.uk

ACKNOWLEDGEMENTS

First and foremost, a very big thank you to Dr Helen Kingston and Jenny Hartnoll. Their common sense and intuitive faith in doing what is right and their trust in each other made it possible for changes to take place both in the town of Frome and in its medical practice. This book would not have been possible without their help and support.

Thanks also go to the senior partners and the staff of Frome Medical Practice, including the kind people of Health Connections Mendip, who have supported the work in spite of hardships of many kinds. Thanks to Professor Allan Kellehear, who has been a tremendous friend and colleague as well as a source of inspiration, for allowing us to use the Compassionate City Charter. His vision and insight provided the source of the term Compassionate Communities and he has spearheaded its development and progress around the world.

Thanks also go to the team at Octopus Books, particularly to Kate Adams who suggested the book in the first place and then provided invaluable feedback to shape it, and to Liz Marvin, who did the hard job of copyediting.

The contributors to the book have all played an invaluable role. Thanks in particular go to Julie Carey-Downes, Jo Trickett, Kathy Fellender for her inspiring story, Sheila Gore and Bewick Abel Thompson.

Julian Abel and Lindsay Clarke

I would like to thank Lindsay Clarke, my dear friend and co-author, who had the difficult job of turning my rough prose into something more readable and interesting. On a more personal level, I would like to thank Carolyn Thompson, my long-suffering partner, who was not only an incredible support both through the time spent working with Frome but also provided invaluable advice about the shape and content of the book. Finally, what I have learned about the power of compassion is due to the kindness of the Khentin Tai Situpa, Akong Rinpoche and Lama Yeshe Rinpoche. Without their patience, compassion and wisdom this book would never have happened.

Julian Abel

INDEX

A

Abel, Julian 93, 112–15, 125, 128, 130–1, 170, 175–6
Abrahams, Patrick 69–70
addictions 35, 48, 58, 108, 164
advertising 33–5
Allah 96
Amnesty International 201
anxiety 17–18, 27, 28, 135, 137, 138, 141–2, 163–4, 175, 177, 190
Apocalypse Now 103
Arab Spring 200
Ardern, Jacinda 203–4
Argentina 187
Aristotle 101
Astley, Neil 103–4
Aujourd'hui 126
Auschwitz 91
Australia 25
auto-immune disorders 134–5
awareness 94–5

B

babies 45
Bachelard, Gaston 103
Bainbridge, Michael 21
befriending services 77, 78–9
Bell, David *Against the Tide* 54–6, 60
Bell, Martin 182–3
bereavement 2, 51, 114, 131, 144, 176, 179, 207, 215, 217
  bereavement counselling 65–7

bereavement groups 70–1, 73, 79, 188
Berlin Wall 200
Bernays, Edward Propaganda 33–4
Bhutan 194
Blake, William 30
blood pressure 43, 48, 123, 136, 159
Brazil 187
Brigham Young University, Utah 42
Buddha, Gautama 90, 96
Buddhism 11, 93
Burke, Edmund 193
Bush, George W. 15
businesses 211–12

C

Cameron, David 15
Canada 187
Capernaum 103
carers 97–8, 113–14
  caring for the chronically ill 120–3
  enhancing networks in times of need 124–9
Carey-Downes, Julie 74
catharsis 101, 103
challenges to compassion 97–100
charities 9, 12
children 38, 45–7, 50–1, 109
  education 163–74
  emotional education 171–3

choirs 114
Christ 96
Chuang Tzu 202–3
civic affairs 185–7
Clarke, Lindsay 121, 169–70
Clinical Commissioning Group
  (CCG), Somerset 20
coeliac disease 134
cognitive behavioural therapy
  (CBT) 98–9
Colombia 187
commerce 33–6
communities 41, 49–51
  building community resources
  78–9
  community connectors 71–5
  community development 80–1
  neo-liberalism 55–6
  participatory community
  development 62–4
  service directories 22–3,
  64–7
  social relationships and human
  health 42–4
  talking cafés 67–71, 79
  trusting the community 58
Community Hospital, Frome 6
compassion 8–12, 206–8
  compassion and self-interest
  195–7
  compassion fatigue 32
  competition and compassion
  51–3
  where did our compassion go?
  28–9
Compassionate City Charter
  186–8, 191, 215–18

Compassionate Communities 5,
  6, 38, 81, 134, 136–7
  approach to healthcare 137–44,
  146, 213–14
  businesses and media 211–12
  civic affairs 185–7
  compassion in education
  163–74, 210–11
  compassion in local government
  180–5
  compassionate organizations
  175–80
  environment 214
  formation of steering committees
  187–91
  lives of individuals 210
  manifesto for compassionate
  communities 209–14
  religion 212
  spreading the word 187
  therapeutic relationship 157–60
  workplaces 175–6, 211–12
Compassionate Frome 7, 12–16,
  39, 40–1, 52–3, 55, 88, 139,
  160, 161–3
  compassionate community
  development 56–9
  hospital admissions 13–14,
  40–2, 57–8
compassionate life 88–9
  facing challenges to our
  compassion 97–100
  meditations to develop
  compassion 95–7
  mindfulness and compassion
  93–5
  power of inspiration 100–5

practising compassion 92–3
recognizing and assessing our
    own resources 90–2
Compassionate Neighbours 78
competition 49, 51–3
Conrad, Joseph *Heart of Darkness*
    103
Coppola, Francis Ford 10
Cornett, Mick 189–90
coronavirus pandemic 205–7
Courtney, Kevin 165

D
Dale, Henry 46
Darwin, Charles 49
De Hennezel, Marie 112
Deguen, Florence 126
dementia 3, 66, 73, 79, 121
depression 17–18, 21, 47, 70,
    108, 133, 135, 139, 141–2,
    163, 201
desperation 27, 58, 109
diabetes 60, 76–7, 79
diet 43, 206
digital revolution 36–8
Dorling Kindersley 59
drinking 43, 206

E
education 163–74, 210–11
Einstein, Albert 136, 167
Eliot, George *Middlemarch* 10,
    102–3
elitism 197–9
Engels, Frederick 31
environment 214
    planetary survival 192–5, 197

ethnic groups 78, 149, 171–3
exercise 43, 63–4, 66
extinction 192–3
Extinction Rebellion 199–201

F
Facebook 129, 187
Facetime 111
fatigue 120–1, 123, 142
Finland 166–7
'flatpack democracy' 29, 180–1
food banks 9, 28
Forster, E M 102
Freud, Sigmund 33
Frome, Somerset 3, 25, 38–9,
    161, 207
    history 19–20, 180
Frome Coffee and Cake
    Bereavement Support
    Group 67
Frome Independent Market 20
Frome Medical Practice 6, 12,
    20–1, 25, 136, 147–8

G
Gandhi, Mahatma 90
GatherMyCrew 129
general practice 133–6
    GPs 17–18, 59–60, 77, 133,
    137, 140–1
    identification of those in need of
    support 146–9
    quality improvement methodology
    151–6
    reorganizing primary care 136–7
    structural changes inside general
    practice 145–6

team meetings 149–51
therapeutic relationship 157–60
Germany 187, 200
Gineste-Marescotti Institute 126
global warming 193
GO FROME 23
Golden Rule 11, 28
Gore, Sheila 183–5, 189
Gotzsche, Peter *Deadly Medicines and Organized Crime* 35
grandparents 50–1
Great War 1914–1918 31–2
Greenpeace 201
Guardian the 17, 133

H
Harlesden, London 21, 58, 62
Hartnoll, Jenny 12, 15, 24–5, 42, 58, 80, 86, 96, 184, 187
  community connectors 71–2, 75
  health trainer 21–4, 61–4
  service directories 22–3, 71
  talking cafés 67–8, 150, 155–6
Harvard Medical School 109
health 42–4
  health coaching 59–60
  health connectors 75–7, 150
  health professionals 42, 75, 115, 118–20
  health trainers 17, 21–2
Health Connections Mendip 12, 59, 63, 80, 85, 86, 161
  community connectors 71–5
  Kathy 81–5
  self-management programme groups 79
  service directory 66–7, 139–40

talking cafés 67–9
Heaney, Seamus 32, 170
heart disease 79
Hein, Piet 182
helping 124–8
  electronic sources of help 128–9
  practical help in the workplace 179–80
Heraclitus 2
Hitler, Adolf 100–1
Holt-Lunstad, Julianne 42–3, 44, 46, 144
homelessness 140, 141
Hoover, Herbert 34
hormones 123, 134, 159
  oxytocin 46–9, 100, 123
hospices 5, 78–9, 130, 175–6, 216
hospital admissions 13–14, 40–2, 57–60, 159
hospital discharges 147–9
housing 65, 139–40

I
identity 107–9
illness 60, 76, 133–6, 186
  caring for the chronically ill 120–3
  Kathy 81–5, 91, 96–7
  supportive networks and ill-health 118–20
  terminal illness 4–5, 125, 128, 176
imagination 100–5
imperial expansion 31
Independents for Frome (IfF) 19, 180–5

indigenous peoples 31
Industrial Revolution 29, 30–31
inflammation 134–5
inspiration 100–5
Institute of Healthcare 137, 152
Insys Therapeutics 35
International Classification of
 Diseases 134
Ireland, Northern 169–70

J
Johnson and Johnson 35
joining forces for compassionate
 change 199–202

K
Kellehear, Alan 186, 215
keraunos 2–7, 84
King, Martin Luther 90
Kingston, Helen 7, 12–15, 24–5,
 43–4, 58, 86, 150
 general practitioner 16–21,
  139–44
knife crime 27, 109, 165
Krause, Nihara 164
Kuan Yin 96

L
Lawrence, D H 104
left-brain thought 36–7
leisure activities 65, 98, 118
Lewis, Benton 101–2
life expectancy 43–4
Lions Club 184
listening support at work 178–9
local government 180–5,
 189–90

loneliness 17, 26–7, 60, 65, 84
 support for the lonely 116–18
longevity 44–6
lung disease 24, 79

M
Macfadyen, Peter *Flatpack
 Democracy* 180–2
Machiavelli, Niccolo 200
macular degeneration 24
Madagascar 100
manifesto for compassionate
 communities 209–14
Marx, Karl 31
McCarthy, Donnachadh *The
 Prostitute State* 197–9,
 201
McGilchrist, Iain *The Master and
 His Emissary* 36
MealTrain 129
media 198–9, 212
meditation 93–5
 meditations to develop
  compassion 95–7
Men's Shed 69–70
mental illness 55, 58, 134, 135
 children 163–4
Mercer, Thomas 193
Merton, Thomas 202
mindfulness 93–5
Moore, Patricia 90
multiple sclerosis 63, 66

N
NASUWT 165
National Education Union (NEU)
 164–5

National Health Service (NHS)
41–2, 59, 71–2, 164
Nelson, Charles *Romania's
Abandoned Children* 109
neo-liberalism 54–6
networks 106–17
  caring for the chronically ill
  120–3
  caring for the dying 130–2
  enhancing networks in times of
  need 124–9
  networks of relationships
  110–16
  social relationships and identity
  107–9
  support for the lonely
  116–18
  supportive networks and ill-health
  118–20
New Zealand 25, 203–4
Next 59

O

OECD (Organisation for Economic
Co-operation and Development)
194
Office of National Statistics
163
Okinawa, Japan 44–5, 51
Oklahoma City, US 189–90
old people 27, 28, 45
online communication 110,
111
Open Age, North Kensington
22
opioid abuse 35
organizations 175–6

developing a compassionate
workplace policy 176–8
listening support in the workplace
178–9
practical help in the workplace
179–80
oxytocin 46–9, 100, 123

P

pain 83–4, 120, 133
palliative care 4–5, 112, 115,
120, 186
Parkinson's disease 66, 79
Parkrun 63–4
Participatory Community
Development 153
pharmaceutical industry 34–5
Pinker, Susan *The Village Effect*
44, 46
planetary survival 192–5, 197
poetry 103–5
Point of Light awards 15
police officers 73, 74
politics 35–6, 55–6
  elitism 197–9
  joining forces for compassionate
  change 199–202
  politics of compassion 202–4,
  212–13
  self-interest 195–7, 202
poverty 29
practising compassion 92–3
Prince's Trust 27
psychotherapy 98–9
Pullman, Philip 30, 39
  The Amber Spyglass 29
Pushkin Trust 169–70

Q

Quakers 30–1
Quality Improvement Methodology
151–6

R

Red Cross 201
refusing help 124–6
relationships 45,47
  inner networks 111–13
  outer networks 113–16
religion 11–12, 28, 188, 209,
  210, 212
residential care 3–4, 125
Resurgence & Ecologist 7
rheumatoid arthritis 81–5, 134
right-brain thought 36
Robinson, Ann 17, 133
Robinson, Sir Ken 166–7, 173
Romania 109, 200
Rotary Club 184
RunDemCrew 118

S

Sacha, Duchess of Abercorn
  169–70
Schopenhauer, Arthur 10–11,
  42
science 36
Second World War 32–3
self-interest 195–7, 202
self-management programme
  groups 79
self-worth 108–9
service directories 22–3, 64–7
Shakespeare, William
  King Lear 102

Romeo and Juliet 103
Sharp, Gene *From Dictatorship to
  Democracy* 199–200
Sinclair, Upton 193
Sinton-Hewitt, Paul 63
Sirolli, Ernesto 152–3
Skype 111
Slack, David 20
slavery 30, 31
Smallbrook Surgery, Warminster
  16–20
smoking 43, 66, 135, 206
social interactions 45–6
social isolation 24, 26, 58, 108,
  133, 207
  illness 60
Social Prescribing 155–6
social relationships 42–4
  identity 107–9
Spain 187
Spencer, Herbert 49
spreading the word 187
St Joseph's Hospice, Hackney
  78
Stark, Hans 91
steering committees 187–91
stem4 163–4
stories 101–3
stress 48–9, 99, 135–6
stroke 3, 24, 40, 69
suicide 17, 58, 112–13, 164

T

talking cafés 67–71, 79, 150–1,
  155–6
Tavistock and Portman NHS Trust
  54

teachers 163–8
technocracy 55–6
technology 36
TED talks 152–3, 167, 173,
    189–90
terminal illness 4–5, 125, 128,
    176
Thatcher, Margaret 54
therapeutic relationship 157–60
Thompson, Abel Bewick 170–4
Thunberg, Greta 199
thyroiditis 134
time-bank schemes 99–100
tobacco industry 34
transport 65
Trickett, Jo 147–8
Twitter 187

U
United Kingdom (UK) 15, 21, 25,
    39, 41, 67, 69, 83, 152, 155,
    160, 187, 198–9
United Nations 192, 197
United States (US) 15, 31, 35,
    198
Universal Declaration of Human
    Rights 1948 159–60
universities 174
University of the Third Age 118

V
Vedanta 11
violence 32, 33
volunteering 91–2
  paid work 99–100
von Eschenbach, Wolfram 102
vows 97–8

W
Wales 187, 191
war 31–3, 202–3
wealth distribution 28–9, 193, 198
Webb, Beatrice 90
weight loss 43, 206
Wesley, John 180
West Side Story 103
WhatsApp 129
Whitehead, A N 30
Woman's Own 54
Women's Shed 69, 70–1
Wordsworth, William 104–5
work 108–9
workplaces 37–8, 175–6,
    211–12
  staff support 176–80
World Health Organization 44

Y
YouGov 27–8
young people 27, 28, 109
  gangs 117–18